The Illustrated Guide to Safe Patient Handling and Movement

Audrey L. Nelson, PhD, RN, FAAN, Director of the Department of Veterans Affairs (VHA) VISN 8 Patient Safety Center of Inquiry, Tampa, FL, has over 31 years of experience in nursing and currently serves as the associate chief of nursing service for research at the Tampa VA, director of the VISN 8 Patient Safety Center of Inquiry, and associate director of research at the University of South Florida College of Nursing. Dr. Nelson has a BSN from the University of South Florida (1977), an MN from Emory University (1980), and a PhD in nursing from the University of Florida (1990). She was appointed by the United States Secretary of Labor to the National Advisory Committee on Ergonomics and served from 2002 to 2004. In 2005, she was awarded the Bernice Owen Award for Research in Patient Care Ergonomics as well as the John Eisenberg Award for Patient Safety and Quality. In 2007, she received the Award of Excellence for Public Health Training from the Centers for Disease Control (CDC), for the Safe Patient Handling Training Program implemented nationally in schools of nursing. She was the editor of a book entitled *Handle With Care: A Practice Guide for Safe Patient Handling and Movement*, published by Springer Publishing in 2006.

Kathleen Motacki, MSN, RN, BC, Lecturer, Henry P. Becton School of Nursing and Allied Health, Fairleigh Dickinson University, has over 30 years of experience in nursing and currently teaches a variety of didactic and clinical courses at the baccalaureate level for students at the 1-year accelerated, 2-year accelerated, 4-year traditional, and RN to BSN levels. She is also a referral liaison at Children's Specialized Hospital, New Brunswick, New Jersey. She holds board certification in pediatric nursing from the American Nurses Credentialing Center (ANCC). She was on the ANCC examination-standard-setting committee for the new pediatric credentialing examination. She obtained her BSN and MSN in transcultural nursing administration from Kean University, Union, New Jersey. She has published several articles in nursing journals, and her first book entitled *Silent Medical Errors* was published in October 2008. As the employee health coordinator at Children's Specialized Hospital, Mountainside, New Jersey, she has served on several committees, including Safety, for which she developed the hospital's safe patient-lifting policy and procedure.

Nancy Nivison Menzel, PhD, RN, PHCNS-BC, COHN-S, CNE, FAAOHN, is an associate professor of community health nursing at the University of Nevada, Las Vegas School of Nursing. Her doctorate is in occupational and environmental health with a research focus on prevention of musculoskeletal disorders (MSDs) in caregivers. She holds three master's degrees—in nursing education, community health, and physiology (occupational health). Dr. Menzel is a certified occupational health nurse-specialist, a certified public health clinical nurse specialist, and a certified nurse educator. She helped to develop the safe patient-handling module for a successful pilot study on changing nursing school curricula, funded by the U.S. National Institute for Occupational Safety and Health (NIOSH) and carried out by the American Nurses Association and the U.S. Veterans Administration's VISN8 Patient Safety Center.

The Illustrated Guide to Safe Patient Handling and Movement

- Audrey L. Nelson, PhD, RN, FAAN
- Kathleen Motacki, MSN, RN, BC
- Nancy Nivison Menzel, PhD, RN, PHCNS-BC, COHN-S, CNE, FAAOHN

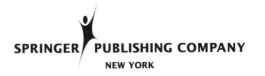

SPRINGER PUBLISHING COMPANY

NEW YORK

Springer Publishing Company, LLC
11 West 42nd Street
New York, NY 10036
www.springerpub.com

Acquisitions Editor: Allan Graubard
Cover design: Steve Pisano
Composition: Monotype, LLC

10 11 12/ 5 4 3 2

Library of Congress Cataloging-in-Publication Data

The illustrated guide to safe patient handling and movement/Audrey L. Nelson, Kathleen Motacki, Nancy Nivison Menzel.
    p. ; cm.
  Includes bibliographical references and index.
  ISBN 978-0-8261-1568-3
  1. Transport of sick and wounded—Handbooks, manuals, etc. 2. Patients—Positioning—Handbooks, manuals, etc. I. Nelson, Audrey, PhD. II. Motacki, Kathleen. III. Menzel, Nancy Nivison.
  [DNLM: 1. Moving and Lifting Patients. 2. Transportation of Patients. 3. Safety Management—methods. WY 100.2 I29 2009]
RT87.T72I65 2009
610.73—dc22

2009002316

Printed in the United States of America by Hamilton Printing

To my husband Robert, my son Robert, my daughter Lisa, my son John, my father-in-law Edward, my mother-in-law Irene, my uncle Ted, and my brother-in-law Brian.

Kathleen Motacki

Contents

Contributing Authors

Andrea Baptiste, MA, OT, CIE, is former manager of the Biomechanics Laboratory and Research Ergonomist at the Tampa VA Patient Safety Center. She is a certified industrial ergonomist and an occupational therapist. She is qualified in medical exercise therapy, functional abilities evaluations, and physical demands analyses. Ms. Baptiste has served as coinvestigator on at least nine funded research projects through VA Health Services Research and Development (HSR&D) and Rehabilitation Research and Development (RR&D) services and has authored more than 16 peer-reviewed publications and completed more than 13 presentations at national conferences. Her research experience includes the evaluation of technologies in the area of patient handling and movement.

Jennifer Giordano, BS, RN, is a nurse in New York City. She has been a bedside clinician, educator and mentor during her 8 years in women's health, preceded by several years of practice in psychiatric nursing. She specialized in labor and delivery, post partum and antepartum care when working as a travel nurse at institutions such as Johns Hopkins Hospital, Stanford University Medical Center, and the University of Pennsylvania. This led her to New York where she now works at the NYU Fertility Center at the NYU Langone Medical Center.

Karen Manning, MSN, RN, CRRN, CNA, is an associate professor at Salem State College in Salem, MA. She is responsible for the planning, development, and evaluation of classroom and clinical instruction for nursing students in the undergraduate program. Her areas of clinical/classroom instruction include rehabilitation nursing, nursing leadership and management, NCLEX preparation, the RN refresher program, and the Direct Entry Master's Program. She also does clinical instruction for the Summer Externship Program. Karen is the 2007–2008 president of the Association of Rehabilitation Nurses.

Patricia Mechan, PT, MPH, CCS, is a physical therapist from Boston, MA. She has over 20 years of experience across a variety of health care settings, including acute care, rehabilitation, and ambulatory care. Patricia has been a bedside clinician, a clinical instructor for students, a team leader, a supervisor, an educator, and an administrative department director. She holds a master's degree in public health and is a board-certified cardiovascular and pulmonary clinical specialist. Patricia is an adjunct faculty member at Simmons College in Boston.

Marylou Muir, RN, COHN, was recently the coordinator of injury prevention and disability management for the Occupational and Environmental Health Unit at the Health Sciences Centre site, the Winnipeg Regional Health Authority, in Winnipeg, Manitoba, Canada. She is now a consultant. The Health Sciences Centre is cross-appointed with the University of Manitoba and is a teaching and research facility. She has assisted in development of the Bariatric Toolkit for the Department of Veterans Affairs (VHA) VISN 8 Patient Safety Center. Ms. Muir has authored several journal articles on the topic of bariatric-patient handling, as well as other ergonomic and occupational health issues. She often teaches educational workshops and speaks internationally.

Laura Murphy, RN, MSN, WHNP, is an OB clinical instructor at Valley Hospital in Ridgewood, NJ. She is responsible for the clinical guidance and teaching of nursing students at Ramapo College in labor and delivery, post partum and nursery. She received a Bachelor of Science in Nursing from the University of Scranton in PA and then began her nursing career as a bedside clinician in labor and delivery at St. Barnabas Medical Center in NJ. She practiced over 7 years at St. Barnabas, a hospital that delivers more babies than any other hospital in NJ, with over 6,000 deliveries a year.

Margaret O'Bryan Doheny, PhD, RN, CNS, ONC, CNE, is a professor of nursing at Kent State University College of Nursing in Kent, OH. Her doctorate is in curriculum and instruction with a focus on nursing and higher education. Dr. Doheny is certified in orthopaedic nursing (ONC) and is a certified nurse educator (CNE). Dr. Doheny is a member of the National Association of Orthopaedic Nursing (NAON) Safe Patient Handling and Movement task force, developed in 2006.

Carol A. Sedlak, PhD, RN, CNS, ONC, CNE, is a professor of nursing at Kent State University College of Nursing in Kent, OH. Her doctorate is in curriculum and instruction with a focus on nursing and higher education. Dr. Sedlak is certified in orthopaedic nursing (ONC) and is a certified nurse educator (CNE). Dr. Sedlak spearheaded the NAON Safe Patient Handling and Movement task force. This task force is working with the ANA, with Dr. Audrey Nelson and colleagues from the James A. Haley Veterans Hospital Patient Safety Center of Inquiry, and with members of the National Institute for Occupational Safety and Health (NIOSH) to prevent work-related musculoskeletal injuries from orthopaedic high-risk tasks.

Linn Steer, PT, works internationally as a clinical advisor and program development manager at the ArjoHuntleigh headquarters in Lund, Sweden. Ms. Steer has worked in international product management and sales/business development since 1998 and has been involved in and responsible for different research and development projects within safe patient handling, hydrotherapy, and hygiene. Apart from physiotherapy and safe patient handling, Ms. Steer has studied architecture and is the editor of the *Arjo Guidebook for Architects and Planners,* which gives advice on how to plan smoothly functioning care facilities.

Elly Waaijer, MSc, CCMM, OT, works internationally as a clinical advisor and program development manager at the ArjoHuntleigh headquarters in Lund, Sweden. She is responsible for developing and supporting intervention programs for safe patient handling. Ms. Waaijer is a certified change management master. For several years she has been responsible for a business unit within Arjo in The Netherlands (Corpus/Diligent) that specializes in safe patient-handling intervention programs. Ms. Waaijer and her Dutch team have developed a complete set of assessment tools and a full training program for ergocoaches and the complete health care staff that includes safe patient-handling guidelines.

Laurette R Wright, RN, MPH, COHN-S, is the Clinical Director of Diligent Services, a division of Arjo, USA. Ms. Wright has practiced in the field of occupational health and safety for 24 years. As clinical director, she manages day-to-day operations and activities of clinical consultants who provide onsite consultation to acute-care and long-term-care facilities throughout the United States. Ms. Wright is an accomplished public speaker and has conducted many presentations and educational offerings on various patient handling and movement topics including peer coaching, competencies within a lifting program, and the safe movement and transfer of the bariatric patient.

Forewords

Without question, the issue of safe patient handling is vitally important. As we progress into a deepening nursing shortage, we must protect our valuable health care resources—our nurses. Nurses and student nurses are at risk for injuries that can impair their health and productivity over both the short and long terms. Nursing consistently ranks in the top 10 occupations with significant work-related musculoskeletal disorders (MSDs), with an average of 7 workdays missed annually as a result.[1] Moreover, as the graying of the nursing workforce continues and as the American obesity epidemic burgeons, MSDs pose great risks not only to individual nurse safety, but also to the retention and recruitment of current and future nurses.[2] As research notes, despite the teaching and implementation of safe patient handling techniques in countless schools of nursing, many nurses still suffer from MSDs. Because safe patient-lifting matrices are complex, staffing shortages continue, and lifting technologies are available, "no-lift" policies must become a research priority for our profession. They must also be part of nursing education as well, even as we make advancements in ergonomics.

Both the American Association of Colleges of Nursing (AACN) and American Nurses Association (ANA) have issued several positions in support of safe patient-handling and no-lift policies. Because many schools have long relied on outdated techniques and approaches to safe patient handling, the ANA supports the introduction of safe patient handling education into the curriculum, including the use of lifting technologies. This effort must also include the sharing of best practices among member institutions in addition to the support of pilot programs focused on safe nursing practice. Because the use and knowledge of safety technologies is critical to safe nurse practice, the AACN and ANA note that, in addition to applying and teaching proper technique and positioning in patient lifting, nurses must also develop the ability to assess and use new technologies. Moreover, as a steadfast advocate for research and evidenced-based practice, the AACN encourages nursing faculty engaged in research to focus on no-lift policies and practices and measure their impact on patient safety.

If we fail to provide our nurses with a safe work environment, I have no doubt that the nursing shortage that currently plagues our country will only intensify.

---

[1] U.S. Bureau of Labor Statistics. (2006). Nonfatal occupational injuries and illnesses requiring days away from work, 2005. Retrieved November 17, 2007 from http://www.bls.gov/news.release/osh2.nr0.htm.

[2] Menzel, N. N., Hughes, N. L., Waters, T., Shores, L. S., & Nelson, A. (2007). Preventing musculoskeletal disorders in nurses: A safe patient handling curriculum module for nursing schools. *Nurse Educator, 32*(3), 130–135.

Not only will advances in technique and the use of no-lift policies utilizing technology create safer work conditions for our nurses, but they will also create safer conditions for our patients. The nursing profession cannot sustain the level of MSDs that it has in the past if it aspires to attract and retain the best and brightest students and professionals. Benjamin Franklin poignantly stated that the definition of insanity was to keep doing what you are doing and expect different results. In regard to safe patient handling, we cannot expect the old ways to generate different outcomes. If we stay the course, we will continue to see alarming rates of MSDs and an assured decline in our workforce, two outcomes that do not bode well for the American health care system. As has been the case in Europe for well over 15 years, we must give serious consideration to collective no-lift policies if we are to protect our nurses and the future of nursing itself.

Jeanette Lancaster PhD, RN, FAAN
Sadie Heath Cabaniss Professor and Dean, University of Virginia
Past President the American Association of Colleges of Nursing

The National League for Nursing (NLN) is proud of the role it has played to support and advance reform in nursing education. The mission of the NLN is to promote excellence in nursing education to build a strong and diverse nursing workforce. The NLN implements it mission guided by four dynamic and integrated core values: caring, integrity, diversity, and excellence. These values permeate the work of the organization to promote the preparation of a nursing workforce that contributes to health care quality and safety. These core values are the foundation of an organization that values the best interests and perspectives of all stakeholders; moves beyond simple tolerance to embrace and celebrate the richness of diverse opinions, systems, and beliefs; and reflects a commitment to continuous growth and transformation.

Within this context, the NLN's current strategic plan calls for enhancing the NLN's national and international impact to become a key player in creating a community of nurse educators from around the world that addresses and influences issues related to excellence in nursing education. This community would also commit itself to being a diverse, member-led organization that champions nurse educators in political, academic, and professional arenas. The advancement of the science of nursing education, through promotion of evidence-based nursing education and the scholarship of teaching, continues to be at the forefront of NLN decision making about future initiatives.

At the forefront of this commitment is recognition that to be a truly effective professional voice for its members, the NLN must create mechanisms to invite dialogue to offer new and differing perspectives. From its earliest days, the NLN has been a catalyst to ignite reform efforts in nursing education. In the 1980s, the NLN supported the leaders of the curriculum revolution and invited nurse educators to be risky and unconventional, to embrace cutting-edge thinking about how teachers teach and how students are taught (Ironside, P., & Valiga, T. M. (2007). How innovative are we? What is the nature of our innovation? *Nursing Education Perspectives, 28*(1), 51–53.). The NLN's position papers on *Innovation in Nursing Education, A Call to Reform* (2003) and *Transforming Nursing Education* (2005) recommended that proposed changes to nursing education be informed by clinical practice and emanate from evidence that substantiates the science of nursing education. Throughout the NLN's history, members of the NLN have called upon their colleagues to be open to new ideas and to rethink approaches to curriculum design.

The authors of this guide to safe patient handling and movement are calling again for reform in nursing education. The movement to create educational environments that promote safe patient-handling techniques will require nurse educators to reframe their thinking, once again, about traditional approaches to body mechanics and to consider new ways to teach tried-and-true, fundamental skills. The evidence-based methods suggested in these pages protect nurses from injury and ultimately improve patient care. The authors seek to create new models for curriculum development and reform, understanding that finding new ways to generate positive and enduring change is the essence of transformation. The NLN is honored to support this essential and pioneering work. These efforts are at the heart of NLN's mission to advance excellence in nursing education to build a competent, ethical, diverse, and caring nursing workforce.

M. Elaine Tagliareni EdD, RN
President, National League for Nursing

Preface

We have over three decades of epidemiological research providing evidence that patient-handling tasks are performed at high risk to the caregiver (Nelson & Baptiste, 2006). In the past decade, technological solutions have emerged to significantly reduce this risk. As with any innovation, it takes time for these new approaches to be imbedded into practice. Changing practice is hard! Nearly every nurse in the United States was taught manual patient-handling techniques during basic training. We now know that there is no safe way to perform manual patient handling (Corlett, Lloyd, Tarling, Troup, & Wright, 1993; Nelson & Baptiste, 2006). The recommended safe limit for manual handling is 35 lbs, a weight far lower than many institutions expect their caregivers to lift routinely (Waters, 2007). Efforts are under way to pass state or national policies banning this practice (Corlett et al., 1993; Hignett et al., 2003; Nelson et al., 2007).

The purpose of this book is to describe new techniques and technologies designed to reduce caregiver risk associated with high-risk patient-handling tasks. A high-risk patient-handling task is defined as any patient-care assignment that pushes the limits of human capabilities, including those that require lifting a heavy load, sustained awkward position, bending/twisting when performing the task, excessive reaching to get the task done, tasks of long duration that contribute to fatigue, tasks that require excessive force on one or more joints or body parts, and tasks that require standing for long periods of time (static posture).

Patient-transfer tasks are high risk and occur in every clinical setting. Chapter 2 describes common patient-transfer tasks that occur across multiple health care settings; these tasks include vertical (seated) transfers, lateral (supine) transfers, bed and chair repositioning, and picking a patient up off the floor after a fall. In addition to these generic high-risk patient-handling tasks, each clinical setting has high-risk tasks that match the patient characteristics and activities unique to that setting. For example, in long-term care settings, over 19 stressful tasks have been identified (Bell, Dalgity, Fennell, & Aitken, 1979; Garg & Owen, 1992; Hui, Ng, Yeung, & Hui-Chan, 2001; Owen, 1987; Owen, Keene, Olson & Garg, 1995; Schibye & Skotte, 2000; Smedley, Egger, Cooper, & Coggon, 1995). Common high-risk tasks in long-term care settings include feeding a resident in bed or a seated position, performing hygiene care in a seated position, and transferring in/out of a geriatric dependency chair.

This book is targeted to meet the needs of students, direct caregivers, managers, administrators, risk managers, educators, industrial hygienists/safety professionals, and researchers of any discipline who are interested in advancing safety for patients and caregivers. Rather than present a generic approach to safe patient handling, this book is one of the first efforts to address not only the commonly encountered high-risk tasks, but also the unique high-risk tasks inherent in specific clinical settings: medical-surgical, critical care, orthopaedics, pediatrics, labor and delivery, rehabilitation, perioperative, and nursing homes (Nelson, 2005). Chapter 3 highlights special risks associated with safe patient handling in morbidly obese (bariatric) patients, whose numbers have increased in all settings.

The science for safe patient handling has evolved. The challenge now is to (1) teach these new evidence-based approaches in schools of nursing, physical therapy, occupational therapy, and other educational programs for direct-care providers; and (2) apply this research to practice in support of safer working environments for caregivers across settings of care. This means eliminating manual patient handling and the over-reliance on body mechanics for safety. Rather, health care settings need to be more focused on evidence-based approaches, including use of patient-handling technologies, environmental modifications, administrative controls (e.g., scheduling, assignments), low-lift policies, clinical decision-making tools (e.g., algorithms or patient-care assessment protocols), staff training on safe use of patient-handling equipment, unit-based peer leaders, or lift teams.

Safe-patient-handling experts from many countries wrote these chapters and provided photographs and video tutorials (on the accompanying DVD) to illustrate techniques. Although the editors ensured that the text reflects best practices, some of the illustrations contain deviations from best practices. You will learn a great deal by comparing "ideal" with "real" on the accompanying DVD. There is also an Instructor's Guide with test questions, available at the Springer Publishing Website.

We know that you will come away from reading this book with information that you can employ in a variety of clinical settings. This is a resource guide that students and instructors can use as a training tool in different clinical rotations, newly hired caregivers can consult to identify patient-handling solutions, and current staff can review for new ways of managing patient care. Opening these issues up for question and resolution in a patient-care environment is an arduous but very rewarding task, and in the end, an essential exercise. Given the looming nursing shortage, implementation of these evidence-based strategies will be a crucial step in recruiting and retaining a competent nursing workforce.

References

Bell, F., Dalgity, M. E., Fennell, M. J., & Aitken, R. C. (1979). Hospital ward patient-lifting tasks. *Ergonomics, 22*(11), 1257–1273.

Corlett, E. N., Lloyd, P. V., Tarling, C., Troup, J. D. G., & Wright, B. (1993). *The guide to handling patients* (3rd ed.). London: National Back Pain Association and the Royal College of Nursing.

Garg, A., & Owen, B. (1992). Reducing back stress in nursing personnel: An ergonomic intervention in a nursing home. *Ergonomics, 35*(11), 1353–1375.

Hignett, S., Crumpton, E., Ruszala, S., Alexander, P., Fray, M., & Fletcher, B. (2003). Evidence-based patient handling: Systematic review. *Nursing Standard 17*(33), 33–36.

Hui, L., Ng, G. Y. F., Yeung, S. S. M., & Hui-Chan, C. W. Y. (2001). Evaluation of physiological work demands and low back neuromuscular fatigue on nurses working in geriatric wards. *Applied Ergonomics, 32*, 479–483.

Nelson, A. L. (2006). Variations in high risk patient handling tasks by practice setting. In A. L. Nelson (Ed.), *Safe patient handling & movement: A practical guide for health care professionals* (pp. 47–58). New York: Springer.

Nelson, A. L., & Baptiste, A. (2006). Evidence-based practices for safe patient handling and movement. *Orthopaedic Nursing, 25*(6), 366–379. Reprinted from *Online Journal of Issues in Nursing, 19*(3), Manuscript 3.

Nelson, A. L., Collins, J., Knibbe, H., Cookson, K., de Castro, A. B., & Whipple, K. L. (2007). Safer patient handling. *Nursing Management, 38*(3), 26–32, quiz 32–33.

Owen, B. (1987). The need for application of ergonomic principles in nursing. In S. Asfour (Ed.), *Trends in ergonomics/human factors IV,* (pp. 831–838). Holland: Elsevier Science Publishers B.V.

Owen, B. D., Keene, K., Olson, S., & Garg, A. (1995). An ergonomic approach to reducing back stress while carrying out patient handling tasks with a hospitalized patient. In M. Hagberg, F. Hoffman, U. Stoessel, & G. Westlander (Eds.), *Occupational health for health care workers*. Landsberg, Germany: ECOMED.

Schibye, B., & Skotte, J. (2000). The mechanical loads on the low back during different patient handling tasks. Proceedings of the IEA2000/HFES 2000 Conference (5, 785–788). Santa Monica, CA: The Human Factors and Ergonomics Society.

Smedley, J., Egger, P., Cooper, C., & Coggon, D. (1995). Manual handling activities and risk of low back pain in nurses. *Occupational and Environmental Medicine, 52*, 160–165.

Waters, T. R. (2007). When is it safe to manually lift a patient? The Revised NIOSH Lifting Equation provides support for recommended weight limits. *American Journal of Nursing, 107*(8), 53–58.

Acknowledgments

Special acknowledgment to Valerie Kelleher for her diligent efforts at editing text and video for the book. Additionally, Linda Smith, RN, and Ehon Hall at the James A. Haley VAMC provided additional support for videotaping miscellaneous tasks missing from various chapters.

The editors and contributors are grateful for the generous financial, equipment, and personnel support for this book from the following companies:

- ARJO, Inc. and ARJO AB
  - Laurette Wright, RN, MPH, COHN-S
  - Amy McCaw
  - Linn Steer
  - Elly Waaijer

- Guldmann, Inc.
  - Patti Mechan, PT
  - Linda Bowman

- Hill-Rom
  - Jan Dubose, RN
  - Brian Wright
  - Melissa Nowitz
  - Dan Gilmore

Chapter 2. Common Patient-Transfer Tasks (Across Multiple Settings)
Thank you to the nursing students at the University of Nevada, Las Vegas and to Antonio Gutierrez, M.S.

We also recognize the kind assistance of the following:

- Department of Occupational and Environmental Safety and Health and the Medical Intensive Care Unit, Winnipeg Health Sciences Centre
- Gail Archer-Heese, O.T. Reg
- Glenn Seroy, Safety Technician

Chapter 3. Bariatric Patient Handling Tasks
The author thanks the following for equipment and facility support:
- Waverley Glen, North America
- Northland Healthcare Products Ltd., Winnipeg, Manitoba

■ MediChair, Winnipeg, Manitoba
■ KCI Medical Group Canada Inc.
■ Calvary Place Personal Care Home, Winnipeg, Manitoba

Thanks to the following for assisting with videos and photos:

■ Matthew Braun O.T.Reg
■ Rose Plessis, RN
■ Jim Mikolajek
■ Bernie Unrau
■ Jon Coutts
■ JoAnn Bunke, Hill-Rom RN

Chapter 4. Medical-Surgical Nursing
Special thanks and acknowledgement to the following individuals for their time and expertise in conducting or editing the videotaping conducted at ARJO, Inc, Roselle, Illinois

■ Wanda Dillberg, RN, Provena St. Joseph Medical Center
■ Donna Hostetler, RN, Diligent Services, ARJO, Inc.
■ Sandra Hough, RN, Diligent Services, ARJO, Inc.
■ Patricia Iroegbu, RN, Diligent Services, ARJO, Inc.
■ Amy McCaw, ARJO, Inc.
■ Andrew Rich, OT/R, Diligent Services, ARJO, Inc.
■ Andy Schneider, Videographer, Digital Take, Chicago, IL

Chapter 5. Critical Care
For survey participation, the chapter authors extend thanks to Registered Nurses from:

■ James A. Haley VA Hospital Critical Care Units—Tampa, FL
■ Oklahoma Heart Hospital PCCU Unit—Oklahoma City, OK
■ Brigham and Women's Hospital Cardiac Surgery ICU—Boston MA
■ Jackson Memorial Hospital South Wing 6—Miami, FL

The authors thank Associate Professor Nancy York of the University of Nevada, Las Vegas School of Nursing for assistance with the case studies.
Additional thanks to the Medical Media Crew at James A. Haley VA Hospital, Tampa, FL, for photo and video support and equipment resource support from Guldmann, Inc.

Chapter 6. Orthopaedics
Special thanks and acknowledgement to the following individuals for their time and expertise in conducting or editing the videotaping conducted at UMass Memorial Medical Center Orthopaedics, Worcester MA:

■ Miki Patterson, PhD, NP, ONC
■ Tony Maciag, Digital Media Specialist

■ Patricia Mechan, PT, MPH, CCS, Guldmann, Inc.
■ Jason Forbes, Media Specialist Kent State University

We also thank the members of the Safe Patient Handling and Movement Task Force in Orthopaedic Nursing—National Association of Orthopaedic Nurses (NAON).

■ National Association of Orthopaedic Nurses (NAON)
  ● Margaret O'Bryan Doheny, PhD, RN, CNS, ONC, CNE
  ● Cynthia M. Gonzalez, MSN, RN, OCNS-C, APN
  ● Cynthia M. Howe, MSN, RN, ONC
  ● Miki Patterson, PhD, NP, ONC
  ● Julia Scaduto, ARNP, MA, ONC
  ● Carol A. Sedlak, PhD, RN, CNS, ONC, CNE

■ National Institute for Occupational Safety and Health (NIOSH)
  ● Thomas R. Waters, PhD, CPE

■ James A. Haley Veterans Hospital, Patient Safety Center of Inquiry
  ● Audrey Nelson, PhD, RN, FAAN
  ● Andrea S. Baptiste, MA (OT), CIE
  ● Valerie Kelleher, AA
  ● John Lloyd, PhD, CPE
  ● Mary W. Matz, MSPH

■ American Nurses Association
  ● Nancy Hughes, MS, RN

■ Guldmann, Inc.
  ● Patricia Mechan, PT, MPH, CCS

■ Diligent Services
  ● Stephanie Radawiec, MHS, PT

Chapter 7. Pediatrics, and Chapter 8. Labor and Delivery

■ Children's Specialized Hospital, New Brunswick, NJ
  ● Trisha Yurochko, Marketing Coordinator
  ● Geri Schuhalter, Nurse Manager
  ● Elaine Mustacchio, Nurse Manager
  ● Robert Motacki, Special Education Teacher
  ● Lisa Motacki, Laundry Aide
  ● John Motacki, Volunteer
  ● Susan Winning, Manager, Physical Therapy
  ● Physical Therapy Department

- Henry P. Becton School of Nursing and Allied Health, Fairleigh Dickinson University, 1000 River Road, Teaneck, NJ
  - Joanne Velarde, Student Nurse
  - Claudette Alfonso, Student Nurse
  - Lois Shallow, Student Nurse

- Guldmann, Inc.
  - Daniel Hedden Photography
  - Patricia Mechan, PT, MPH, CCS

Chapter 9. Patient-Handling Tasks in Rehabilitation
The author thanks Spaulding Rehabilitation Hospital, Boston, MA for the use of their facility and equipment and Patti Mechan, PT, MPH, CCS from Guldmann, Inc. for equipment resource support.

Additional thanks to Salem State College School of Nursing students and Patricia Lyons, Clinical Instructor for their time and help with the video and pictures.

Chapter 10. Nursing Home
We acknowledge the support and assistance of Lena Andersson and Ellen Nilsson at Solhallans Nursing Home, Eslov, Sweden.

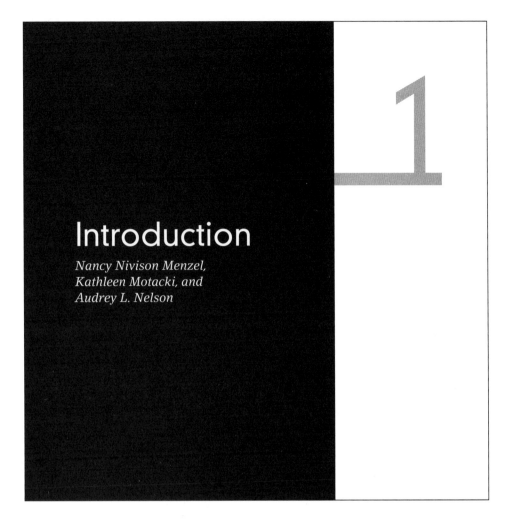

Introduction

Nancy Nivison Menzel,
Kathleen Motacki, and
Audrey L. Nelson

Providing direct patient care is hazardous work. Although a caregiver's risk for infectious disease and chemical exposures are work-related hazards that spring immediately to mind, a less obvious hazard is arguably the most dangerous: manual patient handling. Almost all caregivers face this risk numerous times a day as they provide care to patients who must be repositioned in beds or chairs, transferred from beds and stretchers, transported to various locations in (and out of) health care facilities, assisted with ambulation, and aided in performing the activities of daily living. The risk for caregiver injury has been increased by the rising number of morbidly obese (bariatric) patients seeking health care. In addition to risks to the caregiver, unsafe patient-handling practices can contribute to patient injury, associated with "drops and drags," that is, fall-related injuries during patient transfers or skin tears and lesions associated with sheer force as a patient is pushed/pulled across a surface.

Manual handling has been a job expectation for caregivers since Florence Nightingale's time, despite advances in other industries (e.g., manufacturing and shipping) that rely on technology, not brute strength, to do the heavy lifting. In contrast, hospitals have been slow to adopt new patient-handling technology, relying instead on old-fashioned manual handling.

Schools of nursing, physical therapy, and occupational therapy, both in the United States and internationally, have continued to teach body mechanics, an approach based on the premise that proper body positioning of the caregiver's body will alleviate the damaging forces placed on the musculoskeletal system when performing lifting, turning, and other patient-care tasks. However, there is no evidence that body mechanics alone protect caregivers from the musculoskeletal disorders (MSDs) that result from lifting, repositioning, and moving patients (Hignett, 2003). In fact, the high incidence of MSDs, such as back injuries in caregivers, provides silent testimony to the ineffectiveness of body mechanics in protecting against the forces in a caregiver's normal workload: lifting an estimated 1.8 tons in an 8-hour day (Tuohy-Main, 1997). In 2006, registered nurses had the fifth highest number of MSDs in the United States, exceeding even the traditional laboring occupations of truck driver, construction laborer, and maintenance worker (U.S. Department of Labor Bureau of Labor Statistics, 2007).

In contrast to body mechanics, for which there is no scientific support of effectiveness, there is extensive evidence that supports use of technology for safe patient handling as effective in reducing the strain of lifting heavy loads, frequent repetition of stressful tasks, maintaining awkward postures, standing for long periods of time, bending, stooping, reaching, pushing, and pulling. If schools of nursing, physical therapy, and occupational therapy teach these contemporary, evidence-based approaches, a new generation of graduates will transform the direct caregiving practices; they will view the safety of the caregiver as integral to the safety of the patient and demand technology to protect both parties.

Caregivers who routinely perform unsafe (manual) patient lifting and repositioning are at great risk for MSDs and shortened careers; they then face many years of disability and reduced earnings. Further, the quality of care is jeopardized when care is provided by injured workers who are forced to protect themselves and avoid some patient-handling tasks, or when there are fewer direct caregivers as a result of injured workers. Caregivers can prevent these adverse outcomes by making it their responsibility to know how to work safely in health care.

Understanding Evidence-Based Safe Patient Handling Program

The safe patient-handling program was developed by the Department of Veterans Affairs (VHA) VISN 8 Patient Safety Center of Inquiry (Nelson, 2006b), built on the evidence that the maximum safe manual lift is 35 lb (Waters, 2007). The system is similar to the nursing process, in that it begins with assessing the patient, then goes on to planning and implementation by selecting the most appropriate technique to accomplish the required task. In most cases, these approaches to reduce manual handling require the use of assistive equipment, such as ceiling-mounted patient lifts or friction-reducing devices. In other instances, specialized equipment, such as beds that convert to chairs, eliminate the need for manual handling altogether.

Components of the program, described in more detail by Nelson (2006a), include these:

- Assessment (Assessment Criteria and Care Plan)
- Care Plan (Assessment Criteria and Care Plan)
- Intervention (Algorithms)

Assessment Criteria and Care Plan

Every patient-handling task is different, depending on patient characteristics, condition, and needs. The Assessment Criteria and Care Plan is a caregiver aid to evaluate the patient's upper and lower body strength, ability to understand and cooperate, body mass index (BMI), and the presence of other conditions that affect the patient-handling task. The caregiver uses the assessment criteria to plan the safest way to accomplish the required task. The Assessment Criteria and Care Plan Form is included in Appendix A.

Algorithms

These are step-by-step problem-solving procedures. The algorithms in this book describe the process for carrying out specific patient activities safely. Each algorithm contains a series of decision boxes (based on assessment criteria) to determine the number of caregivers required and the types of equipment that should be used for the designated patient-handling task. An algorithm serves to reduce unnecessary variation in practice and to improve safety outcomes for the caregiver and the patient. The algorithms are guides only; each caregiver must use clinical judgment in selecting or modifying the best approach for an individual patient. The algorithms are included in the Appendices and should be referred to when the text indicates they are applicable. Unfortunately, algorithms do not exist for every high-risk task. In addition to algorithms for common high-risk tasks (originally developed and tested in nursing homes and rehabilitation settings), national task forces in the United States have developed additional algorithms for perioperative care and orthopaedics. Plans are under way to develop and test algorithms in other specialty areas.

Driving Change in Practice by Changing Curricula in Schools of Nursing, Physical Therapy, and Occupational Therapy

In the absence of any national workplace ergonomics standard, many health care facilities have their own policies and procedures on patient lifting and movement. Some may not have any written policies, however, implying that the facility relies on its caregivers to perform tasks in an unsafe manner; that is, manual handling. Facilities may or may not have an adequate number of well-maintained and conveniently located patient-handling assistive devices. Some facilities may have equipment but may not enforce or support its use. If faced with lack of support from their employers, caregivers must speak up to advocate for both themselves and their patients. This book provides the safest approaches to performing many patient-handling tasks; facilities should adopt these approaches as the standard of care.

To help drive change, schools should consider requiring facilities with which they affiliate to provide safe patient-handling equipment. There is evidence that many MSDs begin while a future caregiver is in school and are aggravated in the first year of practice (Klaber Moffett, Hughes, & Griffiths, 1993; Smith & Leggatt, 2004). Schools must become part of the solution and not the origin of the problem.

Further, new graduates should apply for positions only at institutions that provide copies of their safe-lifting policy and a description of the safe-lifting equipment in assigned work areas. In this time of shortages for nurses and therapists, once facilities realize that the new generation of students will be looking for these things upon hire, hospitals may move closer to developing a safe-lifting plan for the facility.

Change is on the horizon. Several U.S. states (e.g., Texas, Washington, Minnesota, Rhode Island) have passed safe patient-handling laws by 2008. The United States lags behind the European Union, which has had regulations that ban manual handling since 1992.

Layout and Use of Book

This book illustrates safe patient-handling and -movement techniques from several different clinical practice settings. It begins with tasks common across all clinical areas, such as transferring a patient from a bed to a chair. It then provides tasks found in specialty clinical areas: bariatrics, medical/surgical, critical care, orthopaedics, pediatrics, labor and delivery, rehabilitation, and nursing homes.

Each specialty chapter is organized as follows:

1. Description of setting
2. Unique challenges to providing safe patient handling in this setting
3. High-risk tasks
4. Objectives
5. Pre-test questions
6. General directions for all tasks
7. Description, risks, assessment criteria, resources, and techniques for each high-risk task identified
8. Case studies with discussion questions
9. Post-test questions
10. References
11. Additional reading

Each chapter includes helpful hints, as well as photographs, illustrations, and video streams depicting the techniques and technologies recommended. Algorithms specify appropriate techniques and technologies, based on patient assessment and task. (Algorithms are clinical tools designed to make an evidence-based decision in a finite number of steps.) Use algorithms as guides only; they do not replace good clinical judgment. Algorithms offer an advantage of reducing unnecessary variations in practice, likely to affect patient and caregiver outcomes. The algorithms are located in the Appendices for easy reference. The Appendices also contain two resource guides: Technology Resource Guide and Sling Resource Guide. The Glossary provides a brief definition of patient-handling terms. Consult the Index to quickly locate tasks you must perform.

Two documents are referred to throughout the book. They are the "Technology Resource Guide" and the "Sling Technology Resource Guide." We did not include them in the book because they are updated regularly, and we wanted to be sure that you had the latest information available.

These guides can be downloaded from the Internet.

- Technology Resource Guide: http://www.visn8.med.va.gov/patientsafetycenter/safePtHandling/default.asp
- Sling Technology Resource Guide: http://www.visn8.med.va.gov/patientsafetycenter/safePtHandling/toolkitSlings.asp

Be sure to read *General Directions for All Tasks* before practicing any of the recommended techniques. This section contains principles and information vital to your safety and the well-being of your patient.

We suggest you begin each chapter by taking the Pre-test to gauge your knowledge of safe patient-handling before reading the techniques. This will help you look for answers while you are reading and looking at the illustrations, so that you will master the post-test questions (which are the same ones).

References

Department of Veterans Affairs (VHA) VISN 8 Patient Safety Center of Inquiry. (n.d.). VISN 8 Patient Safety Center of Inquiry. Web site: http://www.visn8.med.va.gov/patientsafetycenter/.

Hignett, S. (2003). Intervention strategies to reduce musculoskeletal injuries associated with handling patients: A systematic review. *Occupational and Environmental Medicine, 60*(9), E6.

Klaber Moffett, J. A., Hughes, G. I., & Griffiths, P. (1993). A longitudinal study of low back pain in student nurses. *International Journal of Nursing Studies, 30*(3), 197–212.

Nelson, A. L. (2006a). Evidence-based guidelines for patient assessment, care planning, and caregiving practices in safe patient handling and movement. In A. L. Nelson (Ed.), *Safe patient handling and movement: A practical guide for health care professionals* (pp. 59–88). New York: Springer.

Nelson, A. L. (Ed.). (2006b). *Safe patient handling & movement: A practical guide for health care professionals*. New York: Springer.

Smith, D. R., & Leggat, P. A. (2004). Musculoskeletal disorders among rural Australian nursing students. *Australian Journal of Rural Health, 12*(6), 241–245.

Tuohy-Main, K. (1997). Why manual handling should be eliminated for resident and carer safety. *Geriatrician, 15,* 10–14.

U.S. Department of Labor Bureau of Labor Statistics. (2007). Nonfatal occupational injuries and illnesses requiring days away from work, 2006. Retrieved April 10, 2008, from http://www.bls.gov/iif/oshwc/osh/case/osnr0029.pdf

Additional Reading

American Nurses Association. (2007). *Health care worker safety*. Retrieved on April 11, 2008 from http://www.nursingworld.org

Collins, J., & Menzel, N. (2006). Introduction and problem statement. In A. L. Nelson (Ed.), *Handle with care: A practice guide for safe patient handling and movement*. New York: Springer.

Menzel, N., Hughes, N., Waters, T., Shores, L., & Nelson, R. (2007). Preventing musculoskeletal disorders in nurses: Development of a safe patient handling curriculum module for nursing schools. *Nurse Educator, 32,* 130–135.

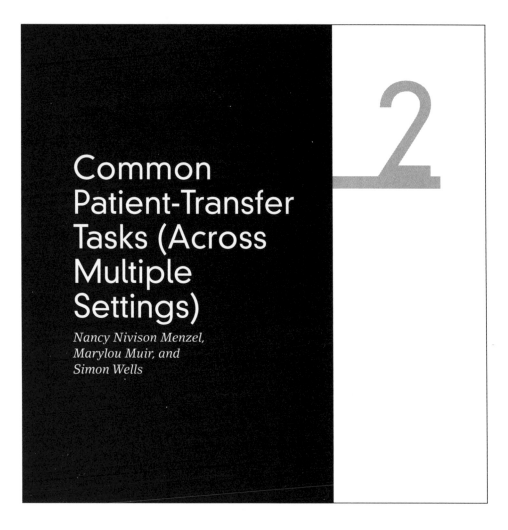

Common Patient-Transfer Tasks (Across Multiple Settings)

*Nancy Nivison Menzel,
Marylou Muir, and
Simon Wells*

Description of Setting

The purpose of this chapter is to familiarize the reader with the principles of patient-handling tasks commonly performed across multiple clinical settings. Subsequent chapters will illustrate tasks associated with specific patient-care areas. In this chapter, we discuss algorithms for patients with a Body Mass Index (BMI) of 50 or lower (Department of Veterans Affairs [VHA] VISN 8 Patient Safety Center of Inquiry, 2006), because larger patients require specialized equipment and procedures due to their body mass and shape. Because each patient has individual needs, caregivers must carefully assess their abilities prior to carrying out any patient-handling or -movement task. Any task requiring the caregiver to lift more than 35 pounds will require the use of patient-handling equipment (Waters, 2007).

Objectives

1. Identify high-risk patient-handling tasks commonly found across many patient-care settings.
2. Delineate the number of caregivers, types of equipment, and techniques for performing each high-risk patient-handling task safely.

Pre-Test Questions

2-1. What is the first step when preparing to handle or move a patient?
    a. Obtain lifting equipment.
    b. Assess the patient.
    c. Select the correct algorithm.
    d. Enlist help of peers.

2-2. What is the most important factor in deciding what technique to use when transferring a patient from bed to wheelchair?
    a. Number of staff available to help
    b. Whether the bed is height adjustable
    c. Patient abilities
    d. Strength of caregiver

2-3. A 145-lb patient, although cooperative, cannot bear weight and has limited upper-extremity strength. If you have to transfer this patient from a bed to a wheelchair, which of these statements is correct?
    a. Three caregivers using good body mechanics will allow for safe manual handling.
    b. A seated transfer aid is appropriate.
    c. Use a gait belt and two caregivers.
    d. Use a floor-based patient lift and two caregivers.

2-4. Mrs. Smith was independent for daily activities. As she was walking to the bathroom, she slipped on some spilled water on the floor and fell to the ground. The nurse found her lying on the floor, trying to get up. The patient is asking the nurse to help pull her up to a standing position. Before assisting the patient up off the floor, the nurse should:
    a. Call for assistance
    b. Cover the patient with a blanket and go for help
    c. Assess the patient for injury and determine the best method to provide assistance
    d. Offer a helping hand and gently pull the patient up off the floor

2-5. Mrs. Smith (described in Question 2-4) can move all her limbs and has a good range of motion but is complaining of a sore shoulder. The nurse should:
    a. Provide a chair and verbal cues for Mrs. Smith to assist herself off the floor
    b. Use a floor-based patient lift to assist her off the floor
    c. Call for three more staff members to manually assist her off the floor
    d. Call for a portable X-ray to examine her shoulder

2-6. Mr. Johnson weighs 225 pounds. He is partially able to assist himself. He has slipped down in bed and needs to be repositioned up and turned on his left side. The nurse should do the following:
  a. Use four caregivers to reposition the patient with draw sheet or incontinence pad.
  b. Without additional caregivers, reposition patient up in bed using a friction-reducing device (FRD) and ceiling-mounted patient lift.
  c. Use two caregivers to reposition the patient using a floor-based patient lift.
  d. Use three caregivers to reposition the patient using an FRD.

General Directions for All Tasks

1. Complete *Assessment Criteria and Care Plan* for patient. Key assessment factors include: physical ability to assist, ability to follow instructions, and cooperation. (Note: weight and height may trigger use of bariatric algorithms.)
2. Review the algorithm for the high-risk patient-handling task to be performed and determine the number of caregivers, types of equipment and techniques for performing each high-risk patient-handling task safely. If no algorithm exists, use the techniques described in this book to guide practice.
3. Check the weight capacity of the equipment to be sure it is safe to handle the patient's weight.
4. Remove obstacles to perform the patient-handling tasks. Obstacles include having too little room to maneuver the equipment, equipment stored on the floor posing a tripping hazard, or inability to perform the activity without threats to patient dignity (e.g., lack of privacy). You may need to remove chairs or bed tables, separate beds, move floor-based equipment, and ask visitors to leave.
5. Make sure selected equipment is in good working order. If the equipment is battery operated, check that the battery is charged. Verify that the appropriate slings and attachments are available. Review safe operation of the equipment, including location of emergency buttons or manual controls in the event of a power failure.
6. Ensure sufficient caregivers are available to help, as specified in the algorithm.
7. Make sure beds are adjusted to caregiver's waist/elbow height before performing bed-related patient-handling tasks.
8. Explain the procedure to the patient and assisting caregivers.
9. Wear gloves according to proper infection-control practices and facility policies.

Patient-Care Slings

A patient-care sling is a fabric device that is used with mechanical lifting equipment to temporarily lift or suspend a patient or body part to perform a patient-handling task. Slings attach to lifts by different types of attachment/

spreader bars. A disposable or patient-specific sling is used for one patient only. Task-specific slings are designed for ambulation, hygiene, limb support, or to support the patient in a standing, supine, or seated position.

- Standing slings assist caregivers to toilet or dress patients, as well as for vertical transfers.
- Supine slings assist caregivers in performing lateral transfers (e.g. transfer in a supine position from bed to stretcher), making occupied beds, bathing, repositioning patients in bed, or rescuing fallen patients from the floor.
- Seated slings enable caregivers to transfer and lift patients in a sitting position, or reposition patients in a chair, among other uses.
- Hygiene slings are made of mesh fabric and are used for showering a patient.

Selecting the right sling for a patient-handling task depends on many factors, including the aim of the task, patient characteristics, and manufacturer's specifications. Caregivers may download a copy of the Patient-Care Sling Selection and Usage Toolkit from the VISN 8 Patient Safety Center of Inquiry for additional information (http://www.visn8.med.va.gov/patientsafetycenter/safePtHandling/toolkitSlings.asp).

Transferring a Patient from Bed to Chair, Chair to Toilet, or Chair to Chair, Using Ceiling-Mounted Patient Lift

Description of Task and Associated Risks

To assist patients to maintain or recover health, vertical patient transfers are needed to transfer from bed to chair (or the reverse). Vertical transfers are performed when the patient is in a seated position. Transferring patients from bed to chair involves the caregiver-risk factors of lifting heavy loads, twisting, awkward postures, and frequency.

Refer to Algorithm 1 (Appendix A). The method required depends on the results of the patient assessment. For patients who are unable to bear weight fully, variations include the use of one of the following: ceiling lift, floor-based patient lift, bed that converts to chair, powered sit-to-stand lift, gait/transfer belt, standing pole, or slide board. This section will address performance of the task using a ceiling-mounted patient lift.

View Video 2.1: Transferring a Patient from Bed to Chair Using a Ceiling Lift

Patient Abilities

- Cannot bear weight
- Either not cooperative or has no upper-extremity strength

Resources Required

A ceiling-mounted patient lift is mounted on tracks above the patient's bed. Some systems allow the patient to be moved throughout the room and into the bathroom, depending on the track layout. Allowing for the length of track, others may permit movement from the bed to a chair or from a chair to a chair. Each system has a different weight limit. Ceiling-mounted patient lift systems have several types of slings that are designed for different purposes, including simple transfers, toileting, and showering. Some slings are disposable (appropriate when infection control is paramount); others must be laundered between patients. Slings are not interchangeable among manufacturers. Major advantages of ceiling-mounted patient lifts over floor-based patient lifts include:

1. Ceiling-mounted patient lifts are conveniently available to caregivers. (Since they are positioned over the bed, one does not need to go find the lift and bring it to the bedside.)
2. The caregiver does not need to work around the base of the lift while performing tasks.
3. Ceiling lifts are quicker to use and do not require additional storage space. Although all have motors to lift or reposition the patient, some also use motors to transport patients along the tracks (power traversing); others depend on the caregiver to manually push/pull the patient along the tracks.

   ■ Ceiling-mounted patient lift with seated sling
   ■ One caregiver (two caregivers needed if patient is uncooperative)

Technique 2-1

1. Follow *General Directions for All Tasks*.
2. Depending on start and end destinations, position the wheelchair, bedside chair, or commode chair next to the bed or position the wheelchair next to the toilet.
3. Select the appropriate sling for the patient. Factors to consider include medical conditions (e.g. spinal fracture, knee or hip injuries, and contractures), purpose of transfer (e.g. toileting, repositioning, bathing, or transporting), patient size, and infection control (disposable vs. reusable).
4. Follow manufacturer's directions for applying the sling. Proper sling positioning is critical for patient safety, dignity and comfort.
5. Attach sling to motor and activate to raise the patient off the bed's surface.
6. Use manual or powered traverse to reposition patient over the chair or toilet, then lower the patient until safe and comfortable contact is made.
7. Depending on the sling design, patient skin integrity, length of time patient will be in the chair or on the toilet, facility policy, manufacturer's recommendations, and the possible need for repositioning—consider leaving the sling in position for a brief period (less than an hour). However, if prolonged contact with the sling material appears likely to compromise skin integrity, remove the sling and keep it nearby for the return transfer.

Transferring a Patient from Bed to Chair, Chair to Toilet, or Chair to Chair, Using Floor-Based Patient Lift

Description of Task and Associated Risks

To assist patients to maintain or recover health through positioning them in a seated position, to help them use the toilet, or to transport them to another area, the caregiver must transfer patients from bed to chair (or the reverse). Transferring patients from bed to chair involves the caregiver-risk factors of lifting heavy loads, twisting, awkward postures and frequency. Patients face the risk of falls or skin shearing.

View Video 2.2: Transferring from Bed to Chair Using a Floor-Based Patient Lift

Refer to Algorithm 1 (Appendix A). The method required depends on the results of the patient assessment. For patients who are unable to bear weight fully, variations include the use of one of the following: ceiling-mounted patient lift, floor-based patient lift, bed that can be profiled to provide a seated position for the patient, powered sit-to-stand lift, gait/transfer belt, standing pole, or slide board. This section will address performance of the task using a floor-based patient lift.

Patient Abilities

- Cannot bear weight
- Either not cooperative or has no upper-extremity strength

Resources Required

Floor-based patient lifts can be moved from room to room. The benefit of this type of patient lift is that it can access the patient in any location, provided there is enough space. Using this type of equipment to lift and transfer patients eliminates the need for caregivers to manually lift. The lift should not be used to transport patients over long distances. Lifts normally feature adjustable leg supports to allow positioning around wheelchairs and special-needs chairs and under most beds. Most lifts have the ability to lift from the floor. The weight limits of the lifts are variable and posted on the lift. Disadvantages include the push/pull forces required to move the lift with the suspended patient to the desired location, potential inconvenient storage far from the patients bed, the need for floor space to accommodate the legs of the lift, and sometimes limited functionality.

- Floor-based patient lift
- One caregiver (two caregivers needed if patient is uncooperative)

Technique 2-2

1. Follow *General Directions for All Tasks*.
2. Depending on start and end destinations, position the wheelchair, bedside chair, or commode chair next to bed or position the wheelchair next to the toilet.

3. Select the appropriate sling for the patient (Department of Veterans Affairs [VHA] VISN 8 Patient Safety Center of Inquiry, n.d.). Factors to consider include medical conditions (e.g. spinal fracture, knee or hip injuries, and contractures), purpose of transfer (e.g. toileting, repositioning, bathing, and transporting), patient size, and infection control (disposable vs. reusable).

4. Follow manufacturer's directions for applying sling. Proper sling positioning is critical for patient safety, dignity, and comfort. Technique to apply sling is usually rolling the patient from side to side. The patient should be positioned supine after sling is inserted underneath him or her.

5. Do not lock the lift's brakes when lifting the patient. The unlocked wheels free the lift to "creep" and maintain the lift's natural center of gravity.

6. Move the lift so that the open end of the base is under the side of the bed or around the base of the chair or commode.

7. Attach loops/clips to lift.

Helpful Hint

Ensure the attachment bar is lowered sufficiently to avoid pulling on or lifting the sling during attachment to the lift.

When transferring the patient consider the position in which you want to transfer him or her; e.g. sitting, semi-recumbent, or supine, and ensure you choose the correct sling and points of attachment to achieve this. If using a sling with loops to achieve a sitting transfer position, use shorter loops at the shoulder and longer at the hip. Always refer to manufacturer's instructions.

8. Instruct patient to cross his or her arms over the chest to ensure the arms remain inside the sling. Operate the controls; raise the patient from the bed to the point of 2–4 inches of clearance from the bed surface. Ensure that the patient is comfortable and that the sling is interfacing with the lift properly.

9. Once the patient is lifted, turn him or her toward the mast (center pole) of the lift. Move the patient to the designated area. If required to ease transport of the lift, adjust its legs.

10. Position the lift directly in front of the chair/toilet, as close as possible. The legs of the lift may need to be adjusted to fit around the chair. Ensure brakes are applied on the wheelchair or commode chair.

11. The first caregiver should maintain eye contact with the patient and ensure a clear view when repositioning the patient, operating the lift controls, and lowering the patient on to the wheelchair or chair. Ensure the patient is facing the mast and not bumping his or her knees. The second caregiver should stand behind the wheelchair or chair to assist in guiding the patient into position.

12. Check manufacturer's recommendations regarding brake application.

13. Lift or lower the patient. When lowering the patient into a chair/toilet, the chair may tip slightly backwards as the patient is lowered; however, this will correct when the patient comes close to the seat pan of the chair. Avoid pulling on the sling.

Helpful Hint

Depending on the sling design, patient skin integrity, length of time patient will be in the chair/toilet, facility policy, manufacturer's recommendations, and the possible need for repositioning - consider leaving the sling in position for a brief period (less than an hour). However, if prolonged contact with the sling material appears likely to compromise skin integrity, remove the sling and keep nearby for the return transfer.

14. Ensure the boom of the lift (the part of the lift that connects the spreader or attachment bar to the mast of the lift) moves slowly away from the patient only after his/her buttocks are in the seat. If the lift is pulled away too soon, the patient will be in a slumped sitting position. If the patient's position is not appropriate, simply raise him/her. Reposition the lift or chair and lower. Do not manually reposition the patient.
15. Detach the sling from the lift. Gently remove the sling from under the patient. Avoid using a stooped posture to remove the sling. Avoid pulling the sling roughly against the patient's skin.
16. To transfer the patient back to the bed or chair, reverse the steps.

Transferring a Patient from Bed to Chair, Using a Bed that Converts to a Chair

Description of Task and Associated Risks

To assist patients to maintain or recover health through positioning them in a seated position, to help them use the toilet, or to transport them to another area, the caregiver must transfer patients from bed to a chair (or the reverse). Transferring patients from bed to chair involves the caregiver-risk factors of lifting heavy loads, twisting, awkward postures, and frequency. Patients face the risk of falls or skin shearing.

View Video 2.3: Chairing the Patient, Using Bed Feature

Refer to Algorithm 1 (Appendix A). The method required depends on the results of the patient assessment. For patients who are unable to bear weight fully, variations include the use of one of the following: ceiling-mounted patient lift, floor-based patient lift, bed that converts to chair, powered sit-to-stand lift, gait/transfer belt, standing pole, or slide board. This section will address performance of the task, using a bed with a feature that allows it to be profiled, forming a chair position.

Patient Abilities

- Cannot bear weight
- Either not cooperative or has no upper-extremity strength

Resources Required

Some beds have the capability to be profiled into a chair position, also known as the cardiac chair position. This type of bed feature assists the patient in sitting upright; the mattress platform is adjusted (profiled) to assist the patient to bend his/her knees, as in a chair-seated position. When the patient requires the health benefits of a seated position, this feature can be used, thus eliminating the need to perform a high-risk patient-transfer task. This bed feature is particularly useful when the patient's tolerance for sitting in a chair is limited (e.g., 10–15 minutes) due to pain, fatigue, illness, or disability.

- A powered bed with "chairing" feature
- One caregiver

Technique 2-3

1. Follow *General Directions for All Tasks*.
2. Ensure the patient is positioned in the center of the bed.
3. Using the bed controls, activate the profiling action "chair bed" feature.
4. Assess the patient for comfort once the desired patient position is achieved.
5. Adjust pillows to provide stability and support for patients who cannot sit unsupported.

Transferring a Patient from Bed to Chair, Chair to Toilet, or Chair to Chair, Using Sit-to-Stand Lift

Description of Task and Associated Risks

To assist patients to maintain or recover health through positioning them in a seated position, to help them use the toilet, or to transport them to another area, the caregiver must transfer patients from bed to a chair (or the reverse). Transferring patients from bed to chair involves the caregiver-risk factors of lifting heavy loads, twisting, awkward postures, and frequency. Patients face the risk of falls or skin shearing.

> View Video 2.4: Transferring a Patient from Bed to Chair, Using a Sit-to-Stand Lift

Refer to Algorithm 1 (Appendix A). The method required depends on the results of the patient assessment. For patients who are unable to bear weight fully, variations include the use of one of the following: ceiling-mounted patient lift, floor-based patient lift, bed that converts to chair, gait/transfer belt, standing pole, slide board, or powered sit-to-stand lift. This section will address performance of the task using a sit-to-stand lift.

Patient Abilities

- Able to partially bear weight
- No hip instability
- Cooperative

Resources Required

A sit-to-stand lift is mobile and battery powered. It can be transported readily and easily. It is designed to encourage patients to participate with the transfers, and it promotes a level of independence when transferring from bed to chair/wheelchair or toilet. The patient is attached to the lift with a sling and is then raised safely and comfortably by operating the controls. The sling used to support this transfer is chosen based on the level of support required by the patient and the task.

- ▪ Sit-to-stand lift
- ▪ Suitable size of sling (follow manufacturer's instructions to identify correct size)
- ▪ One caregiver

Technique 2-4

1. Follow *General Directions for All Tasks.*
2. Assist the patient into a sitting position on the side of the bed, chair, or toilet.
3. Move the lift so that the open end of the base is under the side of the bed or around the base of the chair or commode. Since the patient stands on a platform, the locks must be on.

Helpful Hint

Some beds are provided with mobilization handles that the patient may find useful for holding onto and pushing on and against when standing and, once standing, for support.

Adjust the height of the bed to assist the patient to stand from an optimum height.

If the transfer is in the toilet area, grab bars are often available for the patient to hold on to, for the patient to push on and against when standing, and for patient support when standing.

A standing pole is a device that can be used to help assist patients from sitting to standing, turn them (in standing position), and reposition them on the receiving surface. The aid features a handle that the patient holds and pulls against in order to raise him/herself from sitting to standing, as well as a small, lockable platform on which the patient stands during the transfer. The aid encourages independence and provides support during the transfer.

4. Choose the correct sling and size for the patient's needs. Place the harness/sling around the patient and attach to the lift, ensuring the sling is positioned according to the manufacturer's recommendation. The sling should be snug but need not be tight.

5. Place the patient's arms on the outside of the sling; encourage the patient to hold onto the handrails of the lift.
6. If possible, adjust the kneepad so that the top rests just below the bottom of the patella. The shins should rest into the kneepad. Ensure that the patient's feet are placed in the correct position on the footplate of the lift.
7. Instruct the patient to lean back slightly. If necessary, have him/her look up at you or put a hand on the patient's shoulder as a cue to lean back.
8. Operate the control to raise the patient to a comfortable position. Patients with greater ability to bear weight will be able to tolerate a full standing position. Patients with limited ability to bear weight may not tolerate a full standing position; therefore, adjust accordingly.
9. Adjust the lift legs as required and move the patient to the desired location.
10. Ensure that brakes are engaged on the bed, wheelchair, commode, or dependency chair into which the patient is being transferred. Position the patient to complete the transfer.
11. Lower the patient by pressing the "down" button on the hand-held remote control or on the main operation box on the lift itself. Continue to position the patient while lowering him or her into the receiving chair.
12. Detach sling straps, ensure that feet are off the footrest, move lift away, and remove sling. Provide appropriate support cushions to enable patient to sit supported.

Transferring a Patient from Bed to Chair, Chair to Toilet, or Chair to Chair, Using a Gait Belt

Description of Task and Associated Risks

To assist patients to maintain or recover health through positioning them in a seated position, to help them use the toilet, or to transport them to another area, the caregiver must transfer patients from bed to a chair (or the reverse). Transferring patients from bed to chair involves the caregiver-risk factors of lifting heavy loads, twisting, awkward postures, and frequency. Patients face the risk of falls or skin shearing.

Refer to Algorithm 1 (Appendix A). The method required depends on the results of the patient assessment. For patients who are unable to bear weight fully, variations include the use of one of the following: ceiling-mounted patient lift, floor-based patient lift, bed that converts to chair, gait/transfer belt, standing pole, slide board, or powered sit-to-stand lift. This section will address performance of the task using a gait belt.

Patient Abilities

- Able to partially bear weight
- Able to position/reposition feet on floor
- Able to push down with arms and lean forward
- Able to achieve independent sitting balance
- Fully cooperative and able to follow instructions

Resources Required

A gait belt is a safety device that can be used to help assist and guide a person from one position to another. The gait belt can also be useful to guide a person while walking. Positioning the belt around the patient's waist allows the caregiver to achieve a safer hold on the patient. It can also help decrease the chance of the caregiver hurting his/her back while assisting the patient (assuming it is used correctly, and caregivers consider their body posture and practice good body biomechanics when helping the patient transfer or walk). Although the gait belt provides a handle for the caregiver to hold, gait belts are not designed for lifting the weight of the patient. Always encourage the patient being transferred to assist as much as possible.

There are several kinds of gait belts available. Identify the appropriate size and design required by the patient and the task to be accomplished, taking into account the size and shape of the patient. Gait belts with handles are preferred over belts with no handles because they are easier to use and less stressful on the caregiver.

- Gait belt with handles
- One caregiver

Technique 2-5

1. Follow *General Directions for All Tasks*.
2. Ensure the bed brakes are on to avoid unplanned movement.
3. Move the wheelchair near the bed or toilet (at 90°) without causing an obstruction.
4. Position the gait belt around the patient's waist, ensuring its locking mechanism is secure and comfortable for the patient.
5. Ask the patient to shuffle hips/buttocks forward enough to sit safely on the side of the bed, with feet placed flat on the floor (adjust height of bed as required). Patient's feet should be slightly apart, with one foot in front of the other (walk/stand position).
6. Ask patient to lean forward from the hips.
7. Patient's hands (if possible) should be positioned at sides, ready to push down against the mattress and/or mobilization handles.
8. The caregiver should do one of the following:
    a. *Stand* facing the patient and to the side requiring most support, bend his or her knees, and hold the handling belt with the nearest hand; the other hand supports the back of the patient's shoulder. The caregiver then coordinates the technique with verbal instructions (**"READY – STEADY – STAND"**) and on **"STAND,"** the patient can push down against the mattress/side of bed/mobilization handle/top of the legs while the caregiver stands upright, encouraging the patient forward into a standing position.

Helpful Hint

A slight rocking action by the patient may assist in standing.

b. *Sit* next to the patient, the nearest hand to the patient holding onto the gait belt behind the patient, the caregiver's other hand positioned across the nearest shoulder joint of the patient. (Always consider the maximum safe weight limit of bed.) The caregiver then coordinates the technique with verbal instructions **("READY – STEADY – STAND")** and on **"STAND,"** the patient can push down against the mattress/side of bed/mobilization handle/top of the legs while the caregiver transfers from sitting to standing position, encouraging the patient forward into a standing position.

c. Raise the height of the bed with the patient sitting on the edge of the bed to elevate the patient to a standing position. Ensure he/she is holding on to the mobilization handle or bed safety side rail as the bed is raised.

9. For the options above, the caregiver should transfer his or her weight from one foot to the other during the technique, keeping the back straight, and bending at the hip and knee, using his or her weight and body movement to retain a good posture.

Note: If the patient has suffered a cerebral vascular accident (CVA) and has one weaker side of the body that needs support, the caregiver may consider using standing aids (see below), which reduce the chance of the patient's foot sliding during the transfer. While maintaining contact with the patient by holding the gait belt, guide the patient away from the bed and turn him or her until facing away from the wheelchair.

10. Move the wheelchair forward or have the patient step back until the front edge of the chair is in contact with the back of the patient's knees.
11. Ensure wheelchair brakes are on.
12. Encourage the patient to reach backwards to feel/hold the arms of the wheelchair.
13. Make the patient sit down, with the caregiver bending his or her knees/hips while guiding patient onto the chair.
14. Remove the gait belt.

Transferring a Patient from Bed to Chair, Chair to Toilet, or Chair to Chair, Using Seated Sliding Board

Description of Task and Associated Risks

To assist patients to maintain or recover health through positioning them in a seated position, to help them use the toilet, or to transport them to another area, the caregiver must transfer patients from bed to chair (or the reverse). Transferring patients from bed to chair involves the caregiver-risk factors of lifting heavy loads, twisting, awkward postures, and frequency. Patients face the risk of falls or skin shearing.

Refer to Algorithm 1 (Appendix A). The method required depends on the results of the patient assessment. For patients who are unable to bear weight fully, variations include the use of one of the following: ceiling-mounted patient lift, floor-based patient lift, bed that converts to chair, powered sit-to-stand lift, gait/transfer belt, standing pole, or slide board. This section will address performance of the task using a seated sliding board.

Patient Abilities

- Unable to bear weight on lower extremities
- Stable trunk/sitting balance
- Ability to flex at hips and knees beyond 90°
- Good use of arms

Resources Required

A slide board is a narrow board with a smooth surface acting as a bridge between transfer surfaces. Some patients can use one to slide across from one sitting surface to the next. Slide boards can be useful to promote independence.

- Seated sliding board
- Wheelchair with removable arms
- One caregiver if standby assistance is needed for safety

Technique 2-6

1. Follow *General Directions for All Tasks*.
2. Position wheelchair at 90° to bed/toilet; for bed transfers, adjust height of bed so it is matched with height of wheelchair. Remove wheelchair arm nearest to the bed/toilet.
3. Request patient to transfer weight to position the slide board to bridge gap between the transfer surfaces (refer to manufacturer's instructions on board position); patient to position the board if able.
4. Encourage the patient to bear weight through his or her arms and slide across the board to the receiving surface; this can be completed in small stages. Encourage the patient to move feet (if functionally able) and use upper limbs to gain sideways movement and facilitate the slide. To assist the patient, face the patient, bend knees, and guide the patient through the transfer, moving torso and feet to avoid twisting. Stand by to assist as needed.

Lateral Transfer to/from Bed to Stretcher/Trolley

Description of Task and Associated Risks

Among the most common tasks for caregivers is transferring patients between parallel surfaces; to another; for example, to transfer a patient from a bed to a stretcher in a supine position. Musculoskeletal risks to the caregiver include use of force to push/pull, twisting, awkward postures (from leaning across one of the surfaces), and frequency. Patients are at risk of falls, skin shearing, twisting, and dislodging of medical devices, dressings, or casts.

View Video 2.5: Lateral Transfer to/from Bed Using Sliders

Refer to Appendix A, Algorithm 2. For all but independent patients, this task requires assistive devices.

Factors determining the number of caregivers are patient weight and ability to assist, with three caregivers needed for those over 200 pounds who are unable to assist. Patients may have clinical conditions that require additional caregivers to complete the lift. Examples of such conditions are a leg cast, neck immobilization, central lines, or drainage tubes. Since there are subtle variations in how these devices are used, follow the manufacturer's recommendations for safe use of equipment.

FRDs, also known as sliding sheets, come in several shapes and sizes and are made from different materials with various coatings. Most of the FRDs are nylon based. Their intent and purpose are to reduce the forces caused by friction when repositioning or transferring a patient, thus reducing the exertion needs of the nurse and preventing injuries. They are manufactured as either tubes or flat sheets (most often used in pairs). Some styles incorporate handles or long straps designed to avoid awkward stretching by caregivers across the transfer surfaces when pulling the patient during the lateral transfer.

Patient Abilities

- Partially or not able to assist

Resources Needed

- FRDs
- Lateral transfer board
- One–three or more caregivers, depending on patient's weight, ability to assist, and complicated clinical conditions.

Technique 2-7

1. Follow *General Directions for All Tasks.*
2. Position bed flat (if patient is able to tolerate).
3. Place the FRDs under the patient by rolling the patient from side to side.
4. Place the stretcher and bed side by side. Apply brakes. Ensure that the surface you are transferring to is at the same height as or slightly lower than the starting surface.
5. One caregiver should be positioned at the side of the patient's bed, between the patient's shoulder and hip, the second and third should be positioned at the side of the second transfer surface; between the shoulder and hip and hip lower leg respectively. The caregiver(s) nearest the patient push the patient towards the receiving surface, those positioned opposite pull. Additional caregiver(s) maybe required depending on patient size/weight and ability to cooperate.
6. Position feet in a walking stance. If pushing the patient, shift weight to the front foot during the maneuver. If pulling the patient, shift weight to the rear foot during the maneuver.
7. On a planned count, transfer the patient. Reduce the force exerted and the speed of the transfer because the use of an FRD can significantly reduce friction.

Repositioning in Bed Using FRDs

Description of Task and Associated Risks

Caregivers must reposition patients in bed for a number of reasons, including good nursing practice (to promote circulation and prevent pressure ulcers), patient comfort, respiratory assistance and procedures. Although technology exists to prevent patients from sliding down in bed through the use of specialized beds or nonslip linens, it is not widely available. Risk factors for caregivers include task frequency, push/pull forces, awkward postures, and lifting heavy loads.

View Video 2.6: Repositioning in Bed Using Friction Reducing Device

Refer to Algorithm 4 (Appendix A). This algorithm provides various methods to reposition the patient in bed using equipment, such as FRDs or floor-based or ceiling-mounted patient lifts, depending on patient abilities. The methods of choice have many patient variables, including size, weight, and the number of caregivers available to assist. In addition, the caregiver must consider the patient's pain, level of fatigue, and ability to cooperate. There are several tips included in the algorithm to assist the caregivers. The caregiver must also ensure that other key factors are being addressed such as the bed height, body postures, and communication among all participants during the maneuvers. When patients can assist, coach them to use the side rails and overhead repositioning bars.

Patient Abilities

- Partially able to assist

Resources Needed

- One or two FRDs, depending on patient's ability to assist
- Pillows (one–three) for maintaining the patient in side-lying or tilted positions
- One–three caregivers for a patient ≤200 pounds or three or more caregivers if patient is >200 pounds or uncooperative

Technique 2-8

1. Follow *General Directions for All Tasks*.
   - Position bed flat or, to move patient up in bed, position with head slightly down (if patient is able to tolerate).
2. Ask or assist patient to roll from side to side to place the FRDs underneath patient's head, shoulders, back, and legs.
3. If patient is to be repositioned up in bed, complete the following steps:
   a. Ask or assist patient to roll onto back.
   b. Ask patient to bend the knees and position feet flat on mattress; then tuck chin to chest.
   c. Instruct patient to push into the feet, sliding him/herself up in bed. Provide support for shins if necessary to maximize effort in moving him/herself.

   d. Observe the patient's movement up in the bed. Repeat procedure until patient has reached the desired position in bed.

   e. If patient cannot hold legs in position, the caregiver may provide support. The caregiver supports/holds shins in place during maneuver.

   f. If patient needs more assistance than verbal cuing, position caregivers on each side of the bed. Each caregiver grips (palms up, with wrist rotation neutral if possible) the handles or edge of the uppermost FRD.

   g. With back straight and maintaining a wide base of support, flex knees and hips, and keep elbows close to sides.

   h. One designated caregiver will lead the task; once all are agreed on the commands, the leader communicates the orders to co-ordinate the movement.

   i. Shift weight onto the leg closest to the head of the bed while sliding the patient toward the head of the bed using the upper FRD. Remember, do not twist.

   j. Remove FRDs by asking or assisting the patient to roll from side to side.

4. If patient is to be repositioned on the side, complete the following steps:

   a. Caregiver "A" (facing the direction the patient will face) will pull slightly up and toward self on the FRDs to turn the patient onto his or her side.

   b. Caregiver "B" will assist by placing one hand on the patient's shoulder and one on the hip. "B" will push slightly, moving the patient away.

   c. Caregiver "B" will hold the patient on his or her side by taking the FRD under the raised side of the patient, "A" may then insert pillows behind the patient's back to help support him/her in the required position.

   d. Remove the FRD from under the patient by tucking the FRD under itself and withdrawing diagonally to reduce the potential for the FRD to pull against the patient's skin.

Helpful Hint

To move the patient up in bed, position the bed slightly head down (if patient is able to tolerate).

Repositioning in Bed, Using Ceiling-Mounted or Floor-Based Patient Lift

Description of Task and Associated Risks

Caregivers must reposition patients in bed for a number of reasons, including good nursing practice (to promote circulation and prevent pressure ulcers), patient comfort, respiratory assistance, and procedures. Although technology exists to prevent patients from sliding down in bed through the use of specialized beds or nonslip linens, it is not widely available. Risk factors for caregivers include task frequency, push/pull forces, awkward postures, and lifting heavy loads.

View Video 2.7: Repositioning in Bed Using Friction Reducing Device (Partially Dependent Patient)

Refer to Algorithm 4 (Appendix A). This algorithm provides various methods to reposition the patient in bed using equipment, such as friction-reducing devices or full-body sling lift, depending on patient abilities. The methods of choice have many patient variables, including size, weight, and the number of caregivers available to assist. In addition, the caregiver must consider the patient's pain, level of fatigue, and ability to cooperate. There are several tips included in the algorithm to assist the caregivers. The caregiver must also ensure that other key factors are being addressed, such as the bed height, body postures, and communication among all participants during the maneuvers. When patients can assist, coach them to use the side rails and overhead repositioning bars.

View Video 2.8: Repositioning in Bed Using a Ceiling Lift

Patient Abilities

- Unable to assist

Resources Required

- Ceiling-mounted or floor-based patient lift (Note: Not all floor-based patient lifts are designed to use the sling required for this task.)
- Supine total body sling, hammock sling, or repositioning sling
- Two or more caregivers
- Pillows to maintain patient in side-lying position as required

The ceiling-mounted patient lift and repositioning sling are the preferred equipment combination for this task. A floor-based patient lift can be used but does not interface as well at the bedside for this task. The ceiling-mounted patient lift and rail system minimizes exertion.

Technique 2-9

1. Follow *General Directions for All Tasks.*
2. Lower the head of the bed flat is the patient can tolerate.
3. Apply sling using side-to-side rolling technique. Place the repositioning sling under the patient starting at the top of the head. Some slings are designed to provide extra length; any excess should be at the foot of the bed. If a sling is already in place, assess if its current position is appropriate for use.
4. Ensure a pillow is positioned under the patient's head and shoulders. Position sling attachment bar above and lengthways to the patient.
5. Attach sling to the lift. Ensure the attachment points are attached evenly and equally distributed at each side of the attachment bar. The attachment points are normally at the head, shoulders, hips and lower legs.

Helpful Hint

After a few bed repositions, the repositioning sling may need to be relocated under the patient. The sling will also need replacing when soiled. To replace the sling, it is recommended that the new sling is positioned on the bed while the patient is suspended in the lift in the original sling. Take care when lowering the patient to avoid contamination of the new clean sling.

6. Operating the controls, raise the patient off the bed 2–3 inches. Assess patient tolerance, comfort, and weight distribution in the sling.
7. Slide the ceiling-mounted patient lift along, towards the head of the bed; gently guide the patient's body, lightly pushing against the sling to the desired position. (Some lifts feature powered traverse.)
8. If the patient is to be left in a side-lying position, move the patient along the track to the side of the bed (or move the bed if only a single track system in use)
9. Using the controls, lower the patient on to the bed.
10. Detach straps from one side of the attachment bar only – consider the side to which you are going to turn the patient; maintain the bar lengthways to the patient.
11. Using the controls, raise the bar slightly, using the up button; this will turn the patient onto the side.
12. Position pillows for patient comfort and to maintain position.
13. Lower bar/lift and remove remaining sling straps.
14. Determine whether sling can be left under patient, considering contraindications of skin breakdown and need for frequent assessment of skin tolerance.
15. Do not leave ceiling-mounted patient lift hanging over the patient.

Reposition in Chair: Wheelchair and Dependency Chair

Description of Task and Associated Risks

Patients may slide down in chairs, impairing their ability to breathe and causing strain on their musculoskeletal and circulatory systems. Caregivers must monitor patients to ensure they maintain healthful postures while seated; if they have slid down, caregivers must reposition them in the chair. Risks for caregivers include lifting heavy loads, awkward postures, and frequency. Risks for patients include skin shearing when the sling is removed and being repositioned in an uncomfortable posture.

> View Video 2.9 Patient Repositioning in Dependency Chair

Refer to Algorithm 5 (Appendix A). The type of assistance and equipment needed varies with the patient's ability to assist, bear weight, and cooperate. The caregiver should consider why the patient slipped down and take steps to avoid sliding in the future. For example, some FRDs have one-way textured surfaces that prevent sliding down.

Reclining chairs allow the caregiver to place the patient in a flat position to ease repositioning and then to convert the device into a "chair". There are many types and designs of reclining chairs available; consultation with a therapist may be required to identify a suitable option. The appropriate size and design required by the patient should be identified through assessment and trial and also considering other factors, such as size, shape, weight, condition, and capabilities.

Patient Abilities

- Cannot bear weight
- May or may not be cooperative

Resources Required

- Appropriate Chair
- Floor-based patient lift
- Two or more caregivers (An additional caregiver may be needed if the patient is uncooperative.)
- Optional: one-way FRD (prevents sliding down)

Technique 2-10

1. Follow *General Directions for All Tasks*.
2. If the chair has brakes, ensure they are on to avoid unplanned movement.
3. Position the sling under/behind the patient (referring to manufacturer's instructions).
4. Position the legs/base of the lift under/around the chair (depending on the size of the chair and lift) and lower spreader bar sufficiently to allow easy attachment of the sling to the lift to avoid pulling against the patient when fitting.
5. Attach sling to the spreader bar securely.
6. Operate the lift's control to raise the patient up from the chair. Depending on the size of the patient and lifting height of the lift, it may be necessary to lower the chair (if possible) to ensure clearance beneath the patient and seat of the chair.
7. Position the patient in an upright sitting position. (Some lifts allow adjustment of the patient's sitting position, by repositioning the spreader bar – if available use this feature to ensure the patient is in an upright sitting position in the sling.)
8. Adjust the profile of the chair if possible/as required (e.g., from slightly reclining to upright).
9. Consider positioning a one-way FRD on the seat of the chair (checking manufacturer's instructions on use and positioning).
10. Maneuver the lift so patient can be lowered into correct position on the chair.

11. Position the patient above the chair.
12. Lower the patient onto the chair. It may be useful for one of the caregivers to stand behind/to the side of the chair to guide the patient down onto the chair; the caregiver should avoid pulling on the sling and lifting the weight of the patient when repositioning.
13. Lower sufficiently to allow easy removal of the sling but avoiding collision of the spreader bar and patient.
14. Move the lift away to provide enough room to remove the sling safely from behind/beneath the patient.
15. Remove the legs of the sling from beneath the patient. Encourage the patient to lift his or her legs in order to achieve this. Maintain a good posture when assisting with this task; consider kneeling on the floor to maintain good posture. Never pull the sling against the patient's skin.
16. Sit the patient forward to remove the sling. It may sometimes be appropriate to leave the sling behind the patient to avoid handling when refitting the sling to transfer the patient. Refer to the facility's policy regarding leaving slings in place, as well as the manufacturer's instructions.

Transferring a Patient who has Fallen

Description of Task and Associated Risks

Despite caregiver surveillance and facility safety measures, a patient can fall to the floor. If a caregiver is assisting a patient who falls during ambulation, the caregiver is often injured by reflexively grabbing the falling patient, resulting in excessive forces on the musculoskeletal system. Other risks to caregivers include awkward postures and lifting heavy loads. Risks to fallen patients include musculoskeletal and neurological injuries from ineffective or outdated (manual) rescue attempts.

View Video 2.10: Rescue Fall Patient off Floor with Air-Assisted Device

Refer to Algorithm 6 (Appendix A). This algorithm gives some suggestions to assist patients up off the floor. It is very important for the caregiver properly to assess the patient while the patient is on the floor and not to rush while deciding the appropriate technique to use. Often it takes several minutes to determine the extent of the patient's injuries and capabilities. The patient is safe on the floor. The caregiver should ensure the patient is offered comfort such as a pillow and blanket while appropriate planning occurs.

View Video 2.11: Rescue Fall Patient off Floor with Floor-Based Lift

Patient Abilities

■ Uninjured but unable to assist
■ If patient is injured, seek medical advice before attempting to rescue

Resources Required

- Ceiling-mounted or floor-based patient lift capable of reaching the floor OR air-assisted vertical/lateral transfer device (Note: For use of the ceiling-mounted patient lift, the ceiling tracks need to traverse to the exact location of the patient.)
- Two caregivers (additional caregiver needed if patient is uncooperative)

Technique 2-11

1. Follow *General Directions for All Tasks*.
2. Provide patient comfort and assurance while patient is on the floor; offer pillow and blanket. Position on back, if tolerated.
3. Place the appropriate sling or air-assisted vertical transfer device mattress (with inflatable ports at the feet) under the patient through side-to-side rolling. If using air-assisted lateral transfer device, place sheet or incontinence pads between patient's skin and air mattress. Close safety straps.
4. Approach the patient with the lift base of the support open. Lower the lifting arm to floor level. If using air-assisted vertical transfer device, attach flexible hose end to mattress parallel to foot end and snap in place.
5. Move the patient's legs or head as required to accommodate lift access.
6. Attach the sling to the spreader bar or attach the hose to the air compressor and turn it on to inflate device to desired level for transfer.
7. Raise the patient while constantly observing tolerance, comfort, sling fit, and safety. If concerns arise, lower the patient to the ground immediately.
8. Position patient in chair, stretcher, or bed using the floor-based patient lift or transfer to stretcher or bed using the air-assisted lateral transfer device.
9. Deflate air-assisted device (if used) and then remove either sling or device by rolling patient.

Case Studies

Case Study 2-1

The caregiver is caring for Ms. G, a 78-year-old woman who was transferred from a nursing home to the hospital last night for an emergency appendectomy. The patient's admission notes document the presence of a sacral pressure ulcer. She had a stroke several years ago, leading to right-side paralysis. Owing to the postoperative pain medication she is receiving, she has periods of somnolence. When she is awake, she is cooperative and responsive. The nursing home notes list her height as 5' 4" and her weight as 140 lbs. The physician has ordered her to get out of bed and sit in a chair for 20 minutes three times a day, beginning on the morning that she is assigned to you as a patient. She is in a two-bed room; the other patient has accumulated a large amount of floor-based equipment located between the two beds. The other patient has a large extended family visiting that morning.

Discussion Questions

1. What is the *most important* assessment factor in determining Ms. G's need for assistance in patient handling? Explain your answer.

2. Practice explaining the procedure to the patient with a colleague. Alternately pretend you are Ms. G, critique the clarity and length of each other's explanations.
3. What types of equipment are appropriate for completing this patient-handling task?
4. If the equipment you need is in use for another patient at the moment, what is the best action for you to take?
5. Before beginning the task, what steps would you take based on the environmental assessment?

Post-Test Questions

2-1. What is the first step when preparing to handle or move a patient?
   a. Obtain lifting equipment.
   b. Assess the patient.
   c. Select the correct algorithm.
   d. Enlisting the help of peers.
2-2. What is the most important factor in deciding what technique to use when transferring a patient from bed to wheelchair?
   a. Number of staff available to help
   b. Whether the bed is height adjustable
   c. Patient abilities
   d. Strength of caregiver
2-3. A 145-pound patient, although cooperative, cannot bear weight and has limited upper-extremity strength. If you have to transfer this patient from a bed to a wheelchair, which of these statements is correct?
   a. Three caregivers using good body mechanics will allow for safe manual handling.
   b. A seated transfer aid is appropriate.
   c. Use a gait belt and two caregivers.
   d. Use a floor-based patient lift and two caregivers.
2-4. Mrs. Smith was independent for daily activities. As she was walking to the bathroom, she slipped on some spilled water on the floor and fell to the ground. The nurse found her lying on the floor, trying to get up. The patient is asking the nurse to help pull her up to a standing position. Before assisting the patient up off the floor, the nurse should:
   a. Call for assistance
   b. Cover the patient with a blanket and go for help
   c. Assess the patient for injury and determine the best method to provide assistance
   d. Offer a helping hand and gently pull the patient up off the floor
2-5. Mrs. Smith can move all her limbs and has a good range of motion but is complaining of a sore shoulder. The nurse should:
   a. Provide a chair and verbal cues for Mrs. Smith to assist herself off the floor.
   b. Use a floor-based patient lift to assist her off the floor.
   c. Call for three more staff members to manually assist her off the floor.
   d. Request a portable X-ray to examine her shoulder.

2-6. Mr. Johnson weighs 225 pounds. He is partially able to assist himself. He has slipped down in bed and needs to be repositioned up and turned on his left side. The nurse should do the following:

a. Use four caregivers to reposition the patient with draw sheet or incontinence pad.

b. Without additional caregivers, reposition patient in bed using a friction-reducing device (FRD) and ceiling-mounted patient lift.

c. Use two caregivers to reposition the patient using a floor-based patient lift.

d. Use three caregivers to reposition the patient using an FRD.

References

Department of Veterans Affairs (VHA) VISN 8 Patient Safety Center of Inquiry. (n.d.) *Patient care sling selection and usage toolkit.* Retrieved March 2, 2008, from http://www.visn8.med.va.gov/patientsafetycenter/safePtHandling/default.asp

Department of Veterans Affairs (VHA) VISN 8 Patient Safety Center of Inquiry. (2006). *Safe patient handling and movement algorithms.* Retrieved March 2, 2008, from http://www.visn8.med.va.gov/patientsafetycenter/safePtHandling/default.asp

Waters, T. R. (2007). When is it safe to manually lift a patient? The Revised NIOSH Lifting Equation provides support for recommended weight limits. *American Journal of Nursing, 107*(8), 53–58

Additional Reading

Fell-Carlson, D. (2007). *Working safely in healthcare: A practical guide.* Clifton Park, NY: Delmar Cengage Learning.

Nelson, A. L. (Ed.). (2006). *Safe patient handling and movement: A practical guide for health care professionals.* New York: Springer.

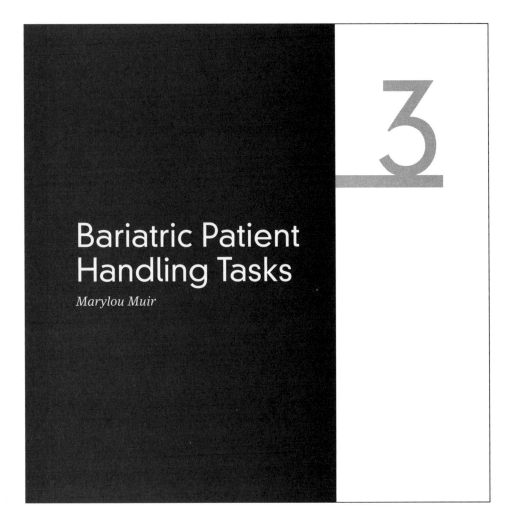

Bariatric Patient Handling Tasks

Marylou Muir

Description of Setting

Caregivers increasingly encounter bariatric (overweight) individuals in all clinical settings. Bariatric patient care can occur on specialized bariatric units or be integrated among many general or specialized care areas, including emergency departments, operating rooms, medical-surgical units, labor and delivery areas, and long-term care.

Unique Challenges to Providing Safe Patient Handling in this Setting

Bariatrics is the science of providing health care to patients who fall into one of these categories:

- Overweight by more than 100–200 lbs
- Body Mass Index greater than 40
- Total weight exceeding 300 lbs

31

Care of bariatric patients presents unique challenges related to promotion of dignity, respect, comfort, and privacy. Patients' medical conditions and physical limitations often limit their ability to function independently in such activities of daily living as hygiene, mobility, and repositioning. Additionally, care of the bariatric patient poses safety risks for the caregiver. The bariatric algorithms are provided to assist you in choosing the correct methods for patient-handling tasks.

High-Risk Tasks

- Transfer to and From Bed/Chair, Chair/Toilet, or Chair/Chair
- Lateral Transfer To and From Bed/Stretcher/Trolley
- Reposition in Bed: Side to Side, Up in Bed
- Reposition in Chair: Wheelchair, Chair, or Dependency Chair
- Patient-Handling Tasks Requiring Access to Body Parts (Limb, Abdominal Mass, Gluteal Area)
- Transporting (Stretcher)

Objectives:

1. Describe the unique challenges associated with safe patient handling in bariatric patient populations.
2. Identify high-risk patient-handling tasks associated with caring for bariatric patients.
3. Delineate the number of caregivers, types of equipment, and techniques for performing each high-risk patient-handling task safely.
4. Compare and contrast weight capacities and ability to accommodate weight distribution of patient-handling equipment.

Pre-Test Questions

3-1. During repositioning of the bariatric patient, the caregiver must consider:
   a. The patient's weight
   b. The size of the bed
   c. The patient's respiratory status
   d. The patient's ability to assist
   e. All of the above
3-2. Bariatric algorithms provide information on which of the following?
   a. The amount of floor space needed to perform the task
   b. The space required in the bed
   c. The number of caregivers required to assist
   d. The patient's medical comorbidities and their relationship to repositioning
3-3. The bariatric patient may be more sensitive to comments and practices of caregivers that impact the patient's dignity. Which of the following might be disrespectful to the patient?

a. Ensuring that there are four people available to assist with a bed boost for a 400-lb patient
b. Posting a sign at the patient's bedside, indicating that because of patient's size, extra precautions are necessary
c. Labeling equipment as extra capacity (EC) with weight designation
d. Asking the patient if he or she would like to consult with the dietician

3-4. Mr. Johnson weighs 410 lbs. He cannot assist in turning from side to side or moving himself up in bed. However, he is cooperative. He has slipped down in bed and needs to be repositioned up and turned on his left side. The nurse should do the following:
a. Using four caregivers, manually reposition the patient up in bed with draw sheet.
b. Using two–three caregivers, reposition patient up in bed and onto his side using bariatric ceiling-mounted patient lift with supine sling.
c. Using two caregivers, reposition the patient up in bed using a floor-based patient lift.
d. Using three caregivers, reposition the patient up in bed using FRDs.

General Directions for All Tasks

1. Complete *Assessment Criteria and Care Plan* for patient. Key assessment factors include: physical ability to assist, and ability to follow instructions and cooperate. Note: weight and height may trigger use of bariatric algorithms.
2. Review the algorithm for the high-risk patient-handling task to be performed and determine the number of caregivers, types of equipment, and techniques for performing each high-risk patient-handling task safely. If no algorithm exists, use the techniques described in this book to guide practice.
3. Check the weight capacity of the equipment to be sure it is able to handle the patient's weight.
4. Remove obstacles to performing the patient-handling tasks. Obstacles include having too little room to maneuver the equipment, equipment stored on the floor and posing a stumbling hazard, or inability to perform the activity without threats to patient dignity (e.g., lack of privacy). You may need to remove chairs or bed tables, separate beds, move floor-based equipment, and ask visitors to leave.
5. Make sure selected equipment is in good working order. If the equipment is battery operated, check that the battery is charged. Verify that the appropriate slings and attachments are available. Review safe operation of the equipment, including location of emergency buttons or manual controls in the event of a power failure.
6. Ensure sufficient caregivers are available to help, as specified in the algorithm.
7. Make sure beds are adjusted to caregiver's waist/elbow height before performing bed-related patient-handling tasks.
8. Explain the procedure to the patient and assisting caregivers.
9. Wear gloves according to proper infection-control practices and facility policies.

Transfer to and from Bed to Chair, Chair to Toilet, or Chair to Chair Using Bed Feature

Description of Task and Associated Risks

To assist patients to maintain or recover health through positioning them in a seated position, to help them use the toilet, or to transport them to another area, the caregiver must transfer bariatric patients from bed to a chair (or the reverse). Transferring patients from bed to chair involves the caregiver-risk factors of lifting heavy loads, twisting, awkward postures, and frequency. Patients face the risk of falls or skin shearing.

View Video 2.3: Chairing the
Patient, Using Bed Feature
(Chapter 2)

Refer to Algorithm 7 (Appendix A). The method required depends on the results of the patient assessment. For patients who are unable to bear weight fully, variations include the use of one of the following: bed that converts to chair, mechanical lifting devices, or sit-to-stand lift. If the nursing goal is to assist the patient to sit, consider using available bed features to perform this task.

Patient Abilities

■ Unable to assist, restricted to bed rest, or non-weight bearing

Resources Required

Some beds have the capability to be positioned into a chairing position. This is often referred to as the cardiac chair position. The feature assists the patient in sitting upright, and the foot of the bed drops down to assist the legs in bending at the knees, as in a chair-seated position. When the patient requires the health benefits of a seated position, the caregiver can use this feature, which reduces or eliminates the physical stress to the caregiver and patient that is associated with the maneuver using other types of equipment. This equipment is of great benefit when the patient's tolerance for sitting is limited by pain, the patient's critical illness requires a short period of time in a chair (e.g., 10–15 minutes), or the equipment (e.g., inappropriate sling fit) or staffing level is not sufficient to enable a safe transfer.

■ One caregiver
■ Powered bed with the remote control ability to position into a seated or cardiac position.

Technique 3-1

1. Follow *General Directions for All Tasks*.
2. Ensure the patient is positioned in the center of the bed.
3. Using the remote control, activate the chair bed feature.
4. Assess the patient for comfort once desired position is achieved.
5. Adjust pillows to provide stability and support for patients who cannot sit unsupported.

Transferring a Bariatric Patient from Bed to Wheelchair Using a Ceiling-Mounted Patient Lift

To assist patients in maintaining or recovering health through positioning them in a seated position, to help them use the toilet, or to transport them to another area, the caregiver must transfer bariatric patients from bed to a chair (or the reverse). Transferring patients from bed to chair involves the caregiver-risk factors of lifting heavy loads, twisting, awkward postures, and frequency. Patients face the risk of falling or skin shearing.

> View Video 3.1: Bariatric Patient Bed-to-Chair Transfer Using a Ceiling Lift

Refer to Algorithm 7 (Appendix A). The method required depends on the results of the patient assessment. For patients who are unable to bear weight fully, variations include the use of one of the following: bed that converts to chair, mechanical lifting devices, or sit-to-stand lift. The algorithm is a guide to help determine the correct technique, but caregivers must use their clinical judgment to determine safety and appropriateness.

Patient Abilities

- Limited or no weight bearing
- Either uncooperative or has limited upper-extremity strength

Resources Required

Ceiling lifts are a type of full-body sling lift that is mounted on tracks above the patient's bed. Some systems allow the patient to be moved throughout the room and into the bathroom, depending on the track layout. Others permit movement only from the bed to a chair or from a chair to a chair. Each system has a different weight limit. Ceiling-lift systems have several types of slings that are designed for different purposes, including simple transfers, toileting, and showering. Some slings are disposable (appropriate when infection control is paramount); others must be laundered between patients. Slings are not interchangeable among manufacturers. Two big advantages of ceiling lifts are their convenient availability to caregivers and their storage out of the way, above the bed. Although all have motors to lift the patient, some also use motors to move patients along the tracks (power traversing); others depend on the caregiver to push the patient along the tracks (manual). The ceiling is preferable for use with the bariatric patient for bed-to-chair transfers because it eliminates the need to move a floor-based patient lift under the load, thus decreasing the exertion required by the caregiver.

- Ceiling-mounted patient lift
- Two caregivers

Technique 3-2

1. Follow *General Directions for All Tasks*.
2. Move chair next to bed.
3. Select the appropriate sling for the patient. Factors to consider include medical conditions (e.g., spine fracture, knee or hip injuries, contractures), purpose

of transfer (e.g., toileting, repositioning, bathing, vertical transfers), patient size and weight distribution, and infection control (disposable vs. reusable).

4. Follow manufacturer's directions for applying the sling, or refer to alternative techniques for sling insertion for the bariatric patient (below).

5. Attach sling to motor and activate it to raise patient off the bed's surface.

6. Use manual or powered traverse to position patient over chair (or toilet); then lower the patient until contact is made.

7. Depending on the sling design, patient's skin integrity, length of time the patient will be in the chair, and the possible need to reposition the patient in the chair, consider leaving the sling in position for a brief period (less than an hour). However, if prolonged contact with the sling material appears likely to compromise patient safety, remove the sling and keep nearby for the return transfer.

Transferring a Bariatric Patient from Bed to Wheelchair Using a Floor-Based Patient Lift

3.1

Bariatric patient transfer using a floor-based lift

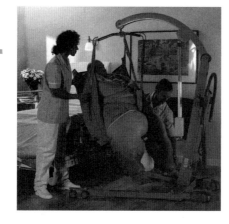

To assist patients to maintain or recover health through positioning them in a seated position, to help them use the toilet, or to transport them to another area, the caregiver must transfer bariatric patients from bed to a chair (or the reverse). Transferring patients from bed to chair involves the caregiver-risk factors of lifting heavy loads, twisting, awkward postures, and frequency. Patients face the risk of falling or skin shearing.

Refer to Algorithm 7 (Appendix A). The method required depends on the results of the patient assessment. For patients who are unable to bear weight fully, variations include the use of one of the following: bed that converts to chair, mechanical lifting devices, or sit-to-stand lift. The algorithm is a guide to help determine the correct technique, but caregivers must use their clinical judgment to determine safety and appropriateness.

Patient Abilities

- Unable to assist
- Uncooperative

Resources Required

Floor-based patient lifts can be moved from room to room. The benefit of this type of patient lift is that it can access the patient in any location, providing there is enough space. Use this equipment to lift and transfer patients, eliminating the need for caregivers to manually lift. The lift is not to be used to transport patients long distances. The lift can fit around wheelchairs and special-needs chairs and under most beds. Most lifts have the ability to lift from the floor. The weight limits of the lifts are variable and posted on the lifts. The lifts are powered and work with a remote control and battery. When using the floor-based patient lift to move a bariatric patient, the load can be very heavy. It is important to plan the move and arrange the work space to prevent having to turn the lift under load. The larger the patient, the more risk there is to the caregivers. Carpeted floors will increase the friction and exertion needed for the caregiver to move the equipment. Whenever possible, the caregiver should use a ceiling-mounted patient lift with sufficient weight capacity instead.

- Floor-based patient lift of sufficient weight capacity
- Minimum of three caregivers

Technique 3-3

1. Follow *General Directions for All Tasks*.
2. Select and inspect the appropriate sling size and type for the patient. Sling selection is based on medical conditions, level of support required, and purpose of the transfer (e.g., toileting sling, transfer sling). A seated-type sling is recommended for this transfer.
3. Follow manufacturer's directions for applying sling. Technique to apply sling is usually rolling the patient from side to side. Patient should be positioned on back after sling is inserted under patient. There is an alternative technique that can be used to insert the sling under the bariatric patient using friction-reducing device (FRD) sheets. See Technique 3-16 for directions.
4. Do NOT lock the brakes when lifting the patient. Unlocked wheels allow them to "creep" and maintain the lift's natural center of gravity.
5. Attach loops/clips to lift. When attaching loops at the shoulders, use the shorter ones to put the patient in an upright-sitting position and longer loops to put patient in a reclining position. When attaching the leg straps of the sling, ensure that the leg pieces fit appropriately and are not causing skin shear to the thighs.

Helpful Hint

Ensure mast (center pole) is lowered enough to ensure you are not pulling on or lifting the sling during attachment to the lift.

6. Instruct patient to cross his or her arms over the chest to ensure arms remain inside the sling. Using the controls, raise the patient 2–4 inches from the bed surface. Ensure the patient is comfortable and the sling is interfacing properly.
7. Lift the patient using the controls and turn the patient toward the mast of the lift.

8. There are two options to place the patient into the chair, depending on the available space:
   a. **Option 1**
      i. Using the provided handles, pull the lift straight back from the bed, moving in one direction, using two caregivers to apply force required.
      ii. Bring the seating device (chair or commode) and place it under the patient in front of the lift, adjusting the chair into position, minimizing the movement of the lift.
   b. **Option 2**
      i. Move the bed away from the area and bring the chair into position, minimizing transporting the patient in the lift.
9. Position the chair directly in front of the patient, as close as possible. Adjust the legs of the lift to fit around the chair. Ensure wheelchair or commode chair brakes are on.
10. One caregiver should position himself or herself behind the mast, using the remote control, and ensuring the patient is facing the mast, not bumping the knees. That caregiver should maintain eye contact with the patient. The second and third caregivers should position themselves behind the wheelchair or chair to assist in guiding the patient into position.
11. Check manufacturer's recommendations regarding brake application.
12. Lower the patient. The chair may tip slightly backwards as the patient is lowered; however, the chair will correct itself when the patient comes close to the seat pan of the chair. Avoid pulling on the sling.
13. Ensure the boom of the lift moves slowly away from the patient only after his/her bottom is in the seat. If it is pulled away before that time, the patient will be in a slumped sitting position. If the patient's position is not appropriate, simply raise him/her. Reposition the lift or chair and lower. Do not manually reposition the patient.
14. Detach the sling from the machine. Gently remove the sling from under the patient. Avoid stooping to remove the sling. Never pull the sling roughly against the patient's skin. The caregiver may insert an FRD between the patient and back of the chair to reduce skin shear and friction during sling removal.
15. The nursing decision as to whether to remove the sling or leave it under the patient should be made with considerations of the patient's skin integrity, tolerance of the sling surface, and length of time in the chair. If the patient is to remain in the chair for an extended period of time or has been transferred to the bed, the recommendation is to remove the transfer sling.

Transferring the Bariatric Patient from Bed to Chair Using a Powered Sit-to-Stand Lift

To assist patients to maintain or recover health through positioning them in a seated position, to help them use the toilet, or to transport them to another area, the caregiver must transfer bariatric patients from bed to a chair (or the reverse). Transferring patients from bed to chair involves the caregiver-risk factors of lifting heavy loads, twisting, awkward postures, and frequency. Patients face the risk of falling or skin shearing.

Refer to Algorithm 7 (Appendix A). The method required depends on the results of the patient assessment. For patients who are unable to bear weight fully, variations include the use of one of the following: bed that converts to chair, mechanical lifting devices, or sit-to-stand lift. The algorithm is a guide to help determine the correct technique, but caregivers must use their clinical judgment to determine safety and appropriateness.

> View 3.2: Bariatric Patient Bed to Chair Transfer Using a Sit-to-Stand Lift

Patient Abilities

- Somewhat able to bear weight
- Able to grip with a minimum of one hand
- Able to maintain a sitting position at the side of the bed

Resources Required

A physiotherapist or other specialist who has been trained in patient assessment must determine if the bariatric patient can tolerate the use of this equipment as it relates to his or her weight-bearing capabilities. The patient size and ability to take weight onto the knee and ankle joint is concerning if there is a limited capacity in one or both legs. This lift has several names; it may also be referred to as a powered-stand assist lift or standing and raising aid. It is portable and battery powered. It can be transported readily and easily in residences and facilities. It is designed to encourage patients to participate with the transfer from bed to chair/wheelchair, or toilet. The patient is attached to the lift with a sling and is then raised by remote control. Choose the sling used to support this transfer based on the level of support required by the patient and the task. Due to limitations of the equipment for bariatric patients for size and fit, it is often better suited to smaller bariatric patients.

- Sit-to-stand lift and sling
- Minimum of two caregivers, based on patient assessment.

Technique 3-4

1. Follow *General Directions for All Tasks*.
2. Assist the patient into a sitting position on the side of the bed.
3. Move the lift so the open end of the base is under the side of the bed or around the base of the chair or commode. Do not engage the locks.
4. Inspect the sling and choose the correct sling and size depending on the patient's size and need for support. Place the harness/sling around the patient and attach to the lift, ensuring the sling is positioned according to the manufacturer's recommendation. The sling should be snug but need not be tight.
5. Place the patient's arms on the outside of the sling and encourage the patient to hold onto the handrails of the lift.

6. Adjust the kneepad so the top rests just below the bottom of the patella. The shins should lean into the kneepad. Ensure that the patient's feet are placed in the correct position on the footplate.

7. Instruct the patient to lean back slightly. If necessary, have the patient look up at you, the operator, or put a hand upon the patient's shoulder as a cue to lean back.

8. Using the remote control up position, raise to the patient's level of comfort. Patients with fuller weight-bearing capabilities will be able to tolerate a full-stand position. Patients with limited weight-bearing capability may not tolerate a full-stand position; adjust accordingly.

9. Adjust the width of the base as necessary. Move the patient straight back and bring the seating device to the patient. If traveling to the bathroom, avoid pivot turns of the lift. Use two caregivers to push the lift. The risk/benefit of moving the patient on the lift must be measured. An option would be to bring the commode chair to the lift.

10. Ensure that brakes are engaged on the wheelchair, commode, or dependency chair into which the patient is being transferred. Position the patient to complete the transfer.

11. Lower the patient by pressing the down button on the handheld remote control or on the main operation box on the lift itself. Continue to position the patient while lowering.

12. If the receiving chair moves slightly into a tipped position, do not be alarmed; the patient is secure. The chair is just adjusting to the center of gravity.

13. Detach straps, ensure that feet are off the footrest, move lift away, and remove sling. Provide appropriate support cushions to enable patient to sit supported.

Lateral Transfer to and from Bed, Stretcher, or Trolley Using Friction-Reducing Devices (FRDs)

Description of Task and Associated Risk

Among the most common tasks for caregivers is transferring patients from one parallel surface to another, for example, from a bed to a stretcher to transport a patient to another location in a supine position. Musculoskeletal risks to the caregiver include use of force to push/pull, twisting, awkward postures (from leaning across one of the surfaces), and frequency. Patients are at risk of falling, skin shearing, twisting, and dislodging of medical devices, dressings, or casts.

Refer to Algorithm 8 (Appendix A). For all but independent patients, this task requires assistive devices. Factors determining the number of caregivers are patient weight and ability to assist, with three caregivers needed for bariatric patients who are unable to assist. Patients may have clinical conditions that require additional caregivers to complete the lift, for example, a leg cast, neck immobilization, central lines, or drainage tubes. Because there are subtle variations in how these devices are used, follow the manufacturer's recommendations for safe use of equipment.

FRDs, also known as sliding sheets, come in several shapes and sizes and are made from different material and coatings. Most are nylon based. Their intent and purpose are to reduce the forces caused by friction when repositioning or transferring a patient, thus reducing the exertion required of the nurse and preventing injuries. They are made in tubes or sheets, often used in pairs. Some styles have long straps designed to avoid awkward stretching across surfaces when pulling the patient across lateral surfaces.

When the patient is bariatric, FRDs must be larger to accommodate for size, and the number of people required to assist with the task may increase. The algorithm recommends FRDs to slide the patient for repositioning side to side or up in bed, as well as for transferring to another surface, such as a stretcher, stretcher chair, exam table or another bed. Often with bariatric patients, FRDs are used to facilitate sling insertion. In order to perform this task, the caregiver must insert the FRDs under the patient. The traditional method requires the patient to roll from side to side, and the FRDs are inserted from the side of the patient using a tuck method. This requires between two and six people, depending on the patient's ability to assist. There are circumstances where the traditional method of insertion cannot work safely due to several issues. Examples would be patient pain and movement intolerance, spinal precautions, mobility restrictions on movement in bed due to fractures, limited bed space restricting the ability to turn the patient onto their side, or not enough staff to assist with the side-to-side method. When this problem arises, the caregiver can use an alternative method of FRD insertion, using an unwrapping technique from head to toe or toe to head. (See Technique 3-16.)

Patient Abilities

- Patient partially able to assist or unable to assist

Resources Required

- Two bariatric-sized FRDs (slippery both sides). Use 1.5 width for patients 400–600 lbs; use double width for patients over 600 lbs
- Two or three caregivers
- Height-adjustable bed with a firm mattress

Technique 3-5

1. Follow *General Directions for All Tasks.*
2. Position bed flat (if patient able to tolerate). Bariatric patients are often unable to tolerate lying flat because of resulting respiratory distress.
3. Place the FRD under the patient by rolling him or her from side to side.
4. Place the stretcher and bed next to each other. Apply brakes. Ensure that the surface you are transferring to is the same height or slightly lower than the starting surface.
5. One or two caregivers should position themselves on the same side of the bed, at the patient's shoulder and hip levels, and one to two caregivers should position themselves at the stretcher side at the patient's shoulder and hip levels. The caregiver(s) on the origination side will push the patient.

6. Position feet in a walk-stance position. If pushing the patient, shift weight to the front foot during the maneuver. If pulling the patient, shift weight to the rear foot during the maneuver.

7. On a planned count, transfer the patient. Reduce the force exerted and the speed of the transfer; the use of an FRD can significantly reduce friction.

Repositioning in Bed: Side to Side, up in Bed With FRDs

Description of Task and Associated Risk

Caregivers must reposition patients in bed for a number of reasons, including good nursing practice (to promote circulation and prevent pressure ulcers), patient comfort, respiratory assistance, and procedures. Although technology exists to prevent patients from sliding down in bed through the use of specialized beds or nonslip linens, it is not widely available. Risk factors for caregivers include task frequency, push/pull forces, awkward postures, and lifting heavy loads.

View Video 2.6: Repositioning in Bed Using Friction Reducing Device (Chapter 2)

Refer to Algorithm 9 (Appendix A). The algorithm for repositioning of the bariatric patient has many of the same principles and equipment used for repositioning of the regular patient. The difference for the bariatric client is that an expanded bed surface may be required to provide the additional space needed to perform the tasks.

This algorithm provides various methods for repositioning the patient in bed using equipment including FRDs. The choice of method depends on patient variables, including size, weight, and the number of people available to assist. Also, the caregiver must consider the patient's pain, level of fatigue, and ability to cooperate. There are several tips included in the algorithm to assist caregivers. The caregiver must also ensure that other key factors are addressed, such as bed height, body postures, and communication among all participants during the maneuvers. Nurses should be sure to coach patients to assist whenever possible by using the side rails and overhead repositioning bars. A ceiling-mounted patient lift and repositioning sling are preferred when available. If not available, use FRDs.

Patient Ability

■ Unable or partially able to assist

Resources Required

FRDs come in several shapes and sizes and are made from different material and coatings. Most are nylon based. Their purpose is to reduce the forces caused by friction when repositioning a patient in the bed, thus reducing the exertion required of the nurse and preventing injuries. They come in tubes or sheets. The method demonstrated below uses two FRD sheets.

- Two FRD sheets
- Two or three caregivers, with additional caregivers to be added for patients over 500 lbs. Consider one additional caregiver for each 100 lbs. of patient weight.
- Pillows for maintaining position patient in side-lying positions (one–three)
- Depending on the patient's capabilities, a repositioning overhead bar may also be an option. Bed side rails may also be of benefit.

Technique 3-6: Positioning Patient up in Bed

1. Follow *General Directions for All Tasks.*
2. Position bed flat after assessing and monitoring the patient's tolerance. When a bariatric patient lies flat, the patient's respiratory condition can be affected. Ensure that if the head is lowered, it is for a minimal time; or consider leaving the head slightly elevated.
3. Roll patient side to side to place the FRDs underneath patient's head, shoulders, back, and legs, or use alternative unwrap Technique 3-16.
4. Roll patient onto back.
5. Each person grips (palms up, with rotation neutral if possible) the handles or edge of the uppermost FRD sheet.
6. Stand on either side of the bed. Maintain a wide base of support, flex knees and hips, and keep elbows close to sides.
7. One designated caregiver will count to three and communicate that the movement will begin on the three count.
8. Shift weight onto the leg closest to the head of the bed while sliding the patient toward the head of the bed.
9. If patient is to move to the side edge of the bed for side repositioning, complete the following steps:
   a. "A" caregivers (facing the direction the patient will face) pull slightly up and toward themselves on the FRDs to tip the patient onto his or her side.
   b. "B" caregivers (on the other side of the bed) will assist by placing one hand on the patient's shoulder and one on the hip on top of the FRD. They will push slightly, moving the patient away from them.
   c. While "B" caregivers hold the patient on the side with the FRD, "A" caregivers will insert pillows to secure the patient in the side-lying position.
   d. Remove the FRDs by pulling diagonally on the underside, starting with the FRD closest to the patient's body.

Repositioning in Bed Using a Ceiling-Mounted or Floor-Based Patient Lift and Repositioning Sling

Description of Task and Associated Risk

Caregivers must reposition patients in bed for a number of reasons, including good nursing practice (to promote circulation and prevent pressure ulcers), patient comfort, respiratory assistance, and procedures. Although technology exists to prevent patients from sliding down in bed through the use of specialized beds or nonslip linens, it is not widely available. Risk factors for caregivers include task frequency, push/pull forces, awkward postures, and lifting heavy loads.

Refer to Algorithm 9 (Appendix A). The algorithm for repositioning the bariatric patient has many of the same principles and equipment used for repositioning the regular patient. The difference for the bariatric client is that an expanded bed surface may be required to provide the additional space needed to perform the tasks.

View 3.3: Bariatric Patient Reposition in Bed Using a Ceiling Lift

This algorithm provides various methods for repositioning the patient in bed using equipment including FRDs. The choice of methods depends on many patient variables, including size, weight, and the number of people available to assist. Also, the caregiver must consider the patient's pain, level of fatigue, and ability to cooperate. There are several tips included in the algorithm to assist caregivers. The caregiver must also ensure that other key factors are being addressed, such as bed height, body postures, and communication among all participants during the maneuvers. Nurses should be sure to coach patients to assist whenever possible, by using the side rails and overhead repositioning bars. A ceiling-mounted patient lift and repositioning sling are ideal when available. If not available, use FRDs.

When using a ceiling-mounted or floor-based patient lift, the patient's size may exceed the lift's weight limit and require an expanded-capacity lift. The slings also may need to be larger and might require a customized sling to fit properly. The sling fit for bariatric patients is difficult due to various patient sizes and shapes. Often facilities are limited in the variation in sizes of bariatric slings. This can contribute to risk of injury to the caregiver and the patient during the transfer. An improper sling fit can cause stress and excoriation, especially in the thigh area. Also, when the patient is in the sling, the tilt of the patient may not line up correctly with the chair. This can put caregivers at risk if they try to adjust and pull on the load manually. A ceiling lift with the repositioning sling is ideal for the bariatric patient. Once the caregiver positions the patient, pillows can provide support to maintain the patient in the desired position. However, in situations where the pillows collapse under the load, wedge-shaped pillows or high density pillows will be required (see Figure 3.1).

Patient's Ability

■ Unable to assist

Resources Required

The ceiling lift and repositioning sling are the preferred equipment combination for this task. A floor-based patient lift can be used but does not interface as well in the environment for this task. Using the overhead lift and rail system to reposition and bed boost is incorporated with a full-body sling, minimizing the caregivers' need for exertion.

- Ceiling-mounted or floor-based patient lift
- Total-body sling, hammock sling, or repositioning sling
- One or two caregivers
- Pillows to sustain patient in side-lying position

Technique 3-7

1. Follow *General Directions for All Tasks*.
2. When possible, apply the repositioning sling to the bed before the patient occupies it. Change slings and bed linens when the patient is suspended in the soiled sling. When no sling is in place, the caregivers apply the sling, using side-to-side rolling technique and right number of people. The initial placement of the sling on the bed requires it to be positioned at the head, with any excess length hanging over foot of bed. If sling is already in place, the caregiver should assess if current sling position and length available are appropriate for use.
3. To attach repositioning sling to lift, lower head of bed flat if patient can tolerate.
4. Ensure a pillow is positioned under the patient's head and shoulders. Position sling attachment bar lengthwise to patient.
5. Attach loop-sling straps to overhead attachment bar on ceiling lift. Ensure the sling loops are attached evenly and equally distributed at each end of the attachment bar. The loops to be attached should be on each side of sling at the positions of the head, shoulders, hips, and lower legs. If using a floor-based patient lift, check with manufacturer if brakes should be applied during the sling attachment.
6. Using the operational controls, raise patient off the bed 2–3 inches. Assess patient tolerance and weight distribution in the sling.
7. Slide the overhead-lift device up toward the head of the bed using the track; gently guide patient's body, lightly pushing on sling to desirable position up in bed. If using floor-based patient lift, reposition the bed to the desirable position under the patient instead of moving the lift.
8. If the patient is to be side-lying, also move the patient using the track to the side of the bed on which he or she will be lying. If using the floor-based patient lift, move it in a straight line forward or backward to position on the side of the bed. (Do not move the lift sideways.)
9. Using the controls, lower patient to bed.
10. Remove straps from sling, maintaining straps on one side of lift, which will assist the patient to turn side-lying. Maintain sling bar lengthwise to patient.
11. Using the controls, raise the lift slightly using the up button; this will turn the patient onto his or her side.
12. Position pillows for patient comfort and to maintain position.
13. Lower lift and remove sling straps.
14. Caregiver identifies whether or not sling can be left under patient, considering such factors as skin breakdown and tolerance.
15. Return floor-based patient lift to charging area.

3.2

Repositioning pillows

Bariatric Reposition in Chair: Wheelchair, Chair, or Dependency Chair

Description of Task and Associated Risks

Patients may slide down in chairs, impairing their ability to breathe and causing strain on their musculoskeletal and circulatory systems. Caregivers must monitor patients to ensure they maintain healthful postures while seated; if they have slid down, caregivers must reposition them in the chair. Risks for caregivers include lifting heavy loads, awkward postures, and frequency. Risks for patients include skin shearing when the sling is removed, and being repositioned in an uncomfortable posture.

Refer to Algorithm 10 (Appendix A). The type of assistance and equipment needed varies with the patient's ability to assist, bear weight, and cooperate. The caregiver should consider why the patient slipped down and take steps to avoid it in the future. For example, some FRDs have one-way textured surfaces that prevent sliding down.

Reclining chairs allow the caregiver to place the patient in a flat position to ease repositioning, then convert back to a chair again. There are many types and designs of reclining chairs available; consultation with a therapist may be required to identify a suitable one. The appropriate size and design required by the patient should be identified through assessment and trial, considering other factors, such as size, shape, weight, condition, and capabilities.

For patients who are unable to assist themselves, caregivers can use the ceiling-mounted or floor-based patient lift to reposition them while they are seated in a chair or wheelchair. The caregiver should also assess why the patient slipped down and how this could be prevented. A proper seating device with appropriate adjustment features, such as a seat tilt, may be helpful. An occupational therapist can assist in identifying the appropriate seating device. Because of the bariatric patient's size, the difficulties of repositioning pose an increased risk. Caregivers should never perform this task manually; the use of equipment or FRDs is imperative. Ideally, the caregiver should use a ceiling-mounted or floor-based patient lift and sling. If the chair can be converted to a stretcher, caregivers should use this feature and FRDs.

Patient Abilities

- Partially able or unable to assist
- Unable to bear weight
- Partially cooperative or uncooperative

Resources Required

- Ceiling-mounted or floor-based patient lift and sling
- FRD
- Three caregivers minimum

Technique 3-8

1. Follow *General Directions for All Tasks.*
2. If feature is available, recline the chair to 45 degrees.
3. With the patient in the upright position, Caregiver 1 should assist the patient in leaning forward slightly.
4. Caregivers 2 and 3 will insert an FRD between the patient and the chair, placing it between coccyx and upper back.
5. Caregivers 2 and 3 will insert the sling between the FRD and back of the chair. The FRD is against the patient to minimize skin shear during insertion of the sling.
6. Insert sling to level of coccyx and remove FRD. Allow patient to sit back into chair (no longer leaning forward).
7. Insert FRD underneath patient's legs, one leg at a time. Pull lift's leg straps gently into place.
8. Align the lift with the patient; if using floor-based patient lift, set the brakes according to the manufacturer's guidelines. Determine if brakes should be on or off during operation and sling attachment.
9. Attach the sling to the lift.
10. Raise the patient from the chair slightly and assess the sling fit and patient's tolerance and comfort. Make adjustments as needed and proceed to lift patient enough to clear the chair (4 inches).
11. Position the patient over the chair:
    a. If using ceiling-mounted patient lift, reposition the patient over the chair into desired position, by gently pushing patient or using the remote controls.

b. If using a floor-based patient lift, move the chair into desired alignment underneath the patient. Caution: Move the chair, not the patient and the lift.
12. Lower the patient into the chair using the controls.
13. Detach the sling from the lift.
14. Remove floor-based patient lift away from the patient.
15. If chair is reclined, raise the chair to upright position.
16. Remove the leg pieces of the sling first, using FRD as described above. Remove the back part of sling using FRDs. Assist the patient in leaning forward.
17. Assess whether patient is secure in chair in desired position.

Patient-Handling Tasks Requiring Access to Body Parts (Abdominal Mass)

Description of Tasks and Associated Risks

The abdominal mass or skin mass on the bariatric patient is also referred to as the pannus. Often caregivers must lift this area in order to access the perineum or abdominal area for tasks such as hygiene care, skin and wound assessment, or catheter insertion. Skin in this area is often in poor condition and can easily tear. The underside of the pannus may also have excoriation, sores, fungal infections, or inflammation. The skin and body can be in a congested state, causing fluid retention, swelling in tissues, and leakage of fluid through the skin. Risk factors to caregivers include reaching, lifting heavy loads, awkward postures, and static load.

Patient Abilities

- Able to assist
- Good upper-arm strength and ability to grasp and lift the pannus

Resources Required

- Flannel sheet or large limb sling
- Two caregivers

Technique 3-9

1. Follow *General Directions for All Tasks*.
2. Fanfold the sheet lengthwise.
3. Place sheet or limb sling under pannus.
4. Instruct patient to hold either end of sheet or ends of sling.
5. Lower head of bed to patient's tolerance level, closely monitoring respiratory status.
6. Instruct patient to hold either end of the sheet/sling and gently pull, raising the pannus while closing monitoring that skin is not being damaged. See Figure 3.3.
7. Provide care to area requiring access, while evaluating patient's tolerance and need for a break from the task. See Figure 3.4.

Patient Ability

- Limited ability to lift the pannus

Resources Required

- Large limb slings or fanfolded flannel sheet
- Three caregivers

Technique 3-10

1. Follow *General Directions for All Tasks*.
2. If using a flannel sheet, fanfold the sheet lengthwise.
3. Position caregivers: one on either side of the bed, facing the foot of the bed.
4. Place sheet/limb sling under pannus.
5. Caregivers should hold either end of sheet or limb sling handles.
6. Lower head of bed to patient's tolerance level, closely monitoring respiratory status.
7. Caregivers gently pull on either end of the sheet/sling and gently raise the pannus, while closing monitoring that skin is not being damaged. See Figure 3.4.
8. Caregivers should maintain a neutral body position for spine and wrists during the tasks.
9. Provide care to area requiring access, while evaluating patient's tolerance. Take breaks as required for comfort of caregivers and patient.

Lifting the pannus

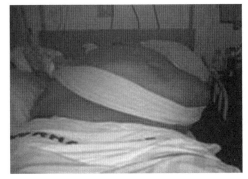

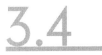

A sling placed under the pannus

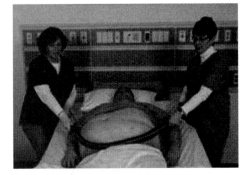

Patient-Handling Tasks Requiring Access to Body Parts (Limbs)

Description of Task and Associated Risks

The following is a description of lifting a bariatric patient's leg for a dressing change. Lifting a patient's leg or holding it for any sustained interval is a task that exceeds safe weight limits. The patient's legs represent 30% of the body

View Video 3.4: Bariatric
Patient—Lifting a Limb for
Dressing Change

weight. Using equipment to perform this task will reduce physical stress for the caregiver and provide comfort for the patient. Risk factors for caregivers include lifting heavy loads, static loads, awkward postures, and reaching.

Patient Ability

- Limited ability to lift and hold leg for dressing change

Resources Required

- Ceiling-mounted or floor-based patient lift
- Limb sling
- One caregiver

Technique 3-11

1. Follow *General Directions for All Tasks.*
2. Preferred patient position is supine; head of bed can be elevated.
3. If task is performed while the patient is sitting in a chair, the caregiver must use a stool or chair to ensure being at the correct working height and preventing bending forward.
4. Place the limb sling under the patient's ankle; this can be facilitated with an FRD.
5. Using the lift device, lift the limb 2–3 inches, observing the patient for comfort. Do not lift beyond the 3 inches because it will cause discomfort to the patient.
6. Perform the dressing change, ensuring the sterile/clean field is maintained during the task. If patient's tolerance is poor, the task may need to be performed in intervals.
   a. Raise leg for removal of the dressing, and assess patients tolerance, lower leg to provide relief from pain if necessary.
   b. Raise leg for cleaning and treatment of the wound and application of clean dressing Continue to assess patient's tolerance and need to lower leg.

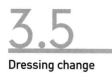

3.5

Dressing change

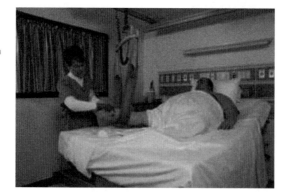

Patient-Handling Tasks Requiring Access to Body Parts (Gluteal Area): Male Catheterization

Description of Task and Associated Risks

Catheterization of both the male and female bariatric patient is complicated by the excess body folds and tissues that obstruct visualization of the urethra. The caregiver must be careful to provide a respectful, private environment while performing this task. Explain the procedure to the patient with specific information as to the need and rationale for any additional staff members. Risk factors for caregivers include lifting heavy loads, sustained awkward postures, reaching, and static load.

Patient Abilities

Most bariatric patients will be dependent and unable to provide assistance for this task. If the pannus is small and the patient is able to provide assistance by lifting and holding it for the required length of time, incorporate this into the task.

Resources Required

- Bariatric limb sling or modified sheet, for use to lift pannus
- Two–four caregivers based on ability to access penis
- Catheterization equipment and supplies

Technique 3-12

1. Follow *General Directions for All Tasks*.
2. Set up all equipment necessary for the male catheterization procedure to ensure that the procedure is not interrupted. Extra catheters and equipment should be accessible at the bedside.
3. Position patient supine; elevate head slightly for patient comfort.
4. Follow the procedure and Technique 3-10 for lifting the pannus to access the groin area.
5. Some patients have additional skin folds in this area that obscure visualization; an additional staff member may be required to retract skin folds to access the penis while the other staff member inserts the catheter.

Patient-Handling Tasks Requiring Access to Body Parts (Gluteal Area): Female Catheterization

Description of Task and Associated Risks

There are several techniques suggested to assist with the catheterization of the female patient. The choices are dependent on the patient's size, ability to assist in maintaining an appropriate leg position, and ability to assume the required positions. The caregiver can access genitalia with the patient in a side-lying position for catheterization or cervical checks during labor. Lying prone, if tolerated, will also provide a position for access. Suspending the patient in a lift with a split-leg sling has provided access. Another option would be using an obstetrical stretcher with leg-support stirrups and a removable foot board. Risk factors for caregivers include lifting heavy loads, sustained awkward postures, reaching, and static load.

Patient Ability

■ Patient is dependent for assistance to support legs or maintain suitable leg position for length of procedure

Resources Required

■ Obstetrical stretcher, one or two caregivers, and a light/lamp stool for caregiver to sit on, or
■ Split-leg sling, one–three caregivers, and a lamp/light, or
■ Patient positioned prone and two caregivers, or
■ Patient positioned side-lying with one-three caregivers assisting

Technique 3-13

1. Follow *General Directions for All Tasks*.
2. Set up equipment for the procedure to ensure adequate and extra supplies are available (e.g., more than one catheter).
3. Position patient:
   a. When using the side-lying technique, the upper leg must be forward and supported. One caregiver will provide assistance in maintaining the leg supported on pillows.
      i. The caregiver would then access the patient from the back.
      ii. One caregiver spreads the buttock cheeks and skin folds and holds them apart while another caregiver performs the procedure.
   b. When using the prone position, the patient can lie semi-prone:
      i. The second caregiver holds the buttocks cheeks apart.
      ii. The labia should be accessible to allow the caregiver to retract them. If the gluteal area is very large, it may be necessary for one caregiver on each side of the patient to pull the folds and cheeks apart. Another caregiver then performs the procedure as per the catheterization protocol.
4. When using the sling and lift device:
      i. Remove the patient's underwear and substitute a gown for this procedure. Ensure the patient is comfortable in the split-leg sling. The patient should be suspended over the bed during the task. Suspend the patient (which is not comfortable) or minimally lift the patient off the bed.
      ii. A second or third caregiver may need to assist in maintaining the skin folds and labia apart to enable the caregiver to view the area and access the urethra.
      iii. Caregiver performs procedure as per protocol.
      iv. Caregiver lowers the patient to the bed as soon as possible.

5. When using the obstetrical stretcher device:
   i. Set up the equipment for the procedure.
   ii. Position patient on the stretcher. (Transfer according to Algorithm 8, Technique 3-4.)
   iii. Remove end of stretcher.
   iv. Position patient's legs on the stretcher leg supports (stirrups).
   v. Set up lighting and stool to enable the caregiver to properly visualize perineal area.
   vi. If required, have second caregiver spread skin folds and labia.
   vii. Complete the procedure per catheterization protocol.

Manual Wheelchair Transport of Bariatric Patient

Description of Task and Associated Risks

When transporting a bariatric patient, consider the following:

- Load of the patient and equipment
- Forces required to push the load
- Pathways and environmental obstacles along the destination
- Possible need for assistance at the destination

Facilities must preplan pathways and routes to various destinations to ensure that doorways and elevators are of appropriate capacity, size, and width. Also, if the route requires transporting over ramps, inclines, and carpeted floor surfaces, facilities must recognize and address the extra forces required. Current technologies provide powered-transport devices that can be attached to beds and wheelchairs. These devices are designed to eliminate the need to manually push or pull. Some motorized-transport devices are independent devices that can be attached to beds or wheelchairs and driven to the destination. Other equipment has for many years had the power drive built in, such as wheelchairs, carts, and scooters. Beds, stretchers, and stretcher-chairs have recently implemented power-drive systems as options for purchase. When planning to care for bariatric patients, consider providing the motorized transport capability to reduce the associated risk of injury. When the need to transport exists and powered equipment is not available, the caregiver should conduct an individual risk assessment on the equipment, patient, and facility to determine the number of people required to manually transport the patient.

For heavier patients, a minimum of two people will be required to push the wheelchair, and a third person may be required to open doors. However, depending on the ease of movement of the wheelchair and the pathway, this may still be an unsafe task. An ergonomic assessment should be completed to determine how much load the wheelchair and two caregivers could safely manage for the destination and task.

Risk factors for caregivers include excessive push/pull forces and awkward postures.

Patient Abilities

- Dependent for transport
- Unable to mobilize long distances
- Transported short distance to eating area, room, or bathroom; not be transported long distances

Resources Required

- Minimum of two caregivers
- Bariatric wheelchair

Technique 3-14

1. Follow *General Directions for All Tasks*.
2. Determine pathway is appropriate in width/height and free of encumbrances for transport.
3. Use powered chair or powered-device attachment if available.
4. If manual chair is being used, choose correct size of chair and weight capacity.
5. Verify that maximum allowable safe push load for caregivers is not exceeded.
6. Ensure patient is properly seated, with feet elevated, and is comfortable.
7. Make appropriate plans for intravenous, oxygen, Foley catheters, and other lines and tubes. Ensure they are safely secured for transport.
8. Using chair, two caregivers push on bar handles on the back of the chair.

Manual Transport of the Patient with Bed or Stretcher

Description of Task and Associated Risks

If transporting a patient in the bed, an ergonomic assessment should determine the number of people required, based on the weight of the patient on the bed. Bed factors such as wheels and steering mechanisms may change the need, with better wheels and steering mechanism reducing the number of caregivers needed. If the situation is urgent and predetermined guidelines have not been developed, consider a rule of thumb of one caregiver per 100 lbs of patient weight to perform the task. Transporting the patient in the bed is often the safest method for both the patient and the caregivers. Current bed designs include the ability of the bed to expand and contract to assist with transport through doorways. Often the patient will need the head of the bed elevated during the transport due to respiratory intolerance related to lying flat. Refer to Algorithm 12 (Appendix A).

Risk factors for caregivers include excessive push/pull forces and awkward postures.

Patient Abilities

- Unable to mobilize to/from destination, either independently or in a wheelchair

- Unable to sit in wheelchair because it is contraindicated
- Undergoing procedures that require patient to be on a bed/stretcher

Resources

- Power-drive support for bed
- Two–three caregivers: one person to operate bed's power, one person to clear pathways and open doors, one person if patient is unstable and requires intensive monitoring during transport

Technique 3-15

1. Follow *General Directions for All Tasks*.
2. Map pathway and identify encumbrances per trip.
3. If using powered bed, stretcher, or transport device, follow manufacturer's recommended procedure for transport.
4. If manual transport, identify required number of people as per Algorithm 12 (Appendix A).
5. If using powered bed, shrink bed if necessary following manufacturer's guidelines.
6. Ensure patient is positioned comfortably for transport.
7. Ensure all tubing and lines are disconnected from wall units.
8. Push bed with two people at head of bed.
9. Place one person at foot of bed to assist with steering, starting, and stopping.
10. Have one person leading in front of bed, opening doors, and clearing the pathway.
11. If additional staff members are required to assist, have them stand at side of bed, using bed frame or rails and applying some assistive pushing force.

Insertion of FRDs Using Alternative Method

Description of Task and Associated Risks

The algorithms recommend FRDs as a method to slide the patient for repositioning side to side or up in bed, or for transferring to another surface, such as a stretcher, stretcher chair, exam table, or another bed. In order to perform the task, the caregiver must insert the FRD under the patient. The traditional method requires that the caregiver roll the patient from side to side and insert the FRDs using a tuck method. This requires two–six people, depending on the patient's ability to assist. There are circumstances when the traditional method of insertion cannot be used. These circumstances include the following: patient pain and movement intolerance, spinal precautions, mobility restrictions on movement in bed due to fractures, or limited bed space restricting the ability to turn a patient onto the side or insufficient staff to assist with the side-to-side method. When this challenge arises, caregivers can use an alternative method of FRD insertion.

Patient Abilities

The patient may be limited in the ability to assist, be dependent, or be partially dependent. The patient may be limited in the ability to assist to roll, or the patient's medical status may make rolling uncomfortable or inappropriate. The patient's cognitive status may also be reduced.

Resources Required

- Two bariatric-sized FRDs (slippery both sides) (Use 1.5 width for patients 400–600 lbs; use double width for patients over 600 lbs.)
- Two caregivers
- Bed with firm mattress

Technique 3-16: Alternative FRD Insertion—Unwrapping Toe to Head

1. Follow *General Directions for All Tasks.*
2. Adjust height of bed to top of iliac crest of the shortest person performing the task.
3. Caregiver places bed flat if patient able to tolerate.
4. Lower side rail, set brakes on bed, and firm mattress (if air loss).
5. One caregiver stands at each side of the bed.
6. Lower side rail, set brakes on bed, and firm mattress (if air loss).
7. Lay FRD on top of patient, with all handles facing ceiling. The end without handles should be just under the patient's chin.
8. Lay second FRD in same position, over top of first FRD. Start folding the FRDs every 4–6 inches.
9. Repeat five to six times, folding the FRDs until all are folded.
10. Grasp folded FRDs; turn FRDs over with folds facing down, away from patient, and insert FRDs under patient's legs.
11. If inserting FRDs over top of the bottom bed sheet, ensure that the bed sheet is pulled tight. It is sometimes appropriate to insert the FRDs against the mattress surface, which reduces binding and catching.

Insertion of Sling—Alternative Method

When the algorithms direct the use of lift equipment, the caregiver must insert a sling under the patient. This technique can be used for every type of sling, including split-leg sling, hammock sling, repositioning sling, etc. Insertion of the sling can be a very difficult task with a bariatric patient; the traditional method of sling insertion requires the patient to roll from side to side, either independently or with assistance. In situations where this traditional method cannot be used (limitations in the number of staff, too small a bed space, or inability to move the patient due to pain or medical condition), an alternative method is recommended. This method is insertion from the head between two FRDs. Risk factors for caregivers include push/pull exertion and awkward postures.

Patient Abilities

- The patient may be able to assist and should be instructed to do so to facilitate this task. If the patient is dependent and limited in the ability to assist, this is also an appropriate method.

Resources Required

- Two FRDs (slippery both sides and bariatric sized) (Use 1.5 widths for patients 400–600 lbs, and use double width for patients over 600 lbs.)
- One bariatric sling
- Two caregivers

Technique 3-17: Alternative Sling-Insertion Method for Supine Patients Unable to Roll FRDs must already be in place

1. Follow *General Directions for All Tasks*.
2. Ensure bed brakes are on; lower head of bed and flatten knee area if elevated.
3. Lower side rails, if the mattress has lost air, put on firm mode for the task.
4. Ensure FRDs are in place.
5. Once FRDs are in place, take sling (assuming it has been assessed for fit) and insert under the head and shoulders of patient between the FRDs.
6. If the patient can assist, cue the patient to adjust his or her body by leaning forward to ease the insertion of the sling between the FRDs.
7. Head: Place lower half of sling between two FRDs. Line up pleats with patient's spine and pull lower half of sling between FRDs, toward patient's feet, to correct position. Hold top FRD taut while pulling sling.
8. Remove upper FRD by passing bottom corner underneath to opposite staff member and gently pulling, as per technique demonstrated in FRD insertion and removal.

Case Study 3-1

Mr. H weighs 500 lbs and is scheduled for spinal surgery. Currently, he can ambulate and reposition himself within the bed. However, after his surgery he will be dependent for repositioning for 24–48 hours. He will need to be transported to the pre-op room, the operating room, the recovery room, and then back to his room on his unit the day of surgery. He has a leg ulcer that requires daily dressing changes. The bed provided does not have power drive but one is available; also in the past a power-drive hookup has been used to move the existing bed. He will need catheterization prior to his surgery in the pre-op area. On Day 2, Mr. H has been cleared to sit in a bedside chair but does not have the strength in his legs to transfer. You will use the ceiling lift and transfer sling to transfer him to his chair. Prior to surgery you were able to try the bed, FRDs, wheelchair, and stretcher to determine the patient's comfort level. Also, the patient had pre-op teaching in ambulating and repositioning in bed using the techniques that he will use after his surgery.

Discussion Questions:

1. As the caregiver assigned to Mr. H, you will need to coordinate his repositioning in bed postoperatively. What are appropriate choices and techniques?
2. What is the best way to transport Mr. H to the perioperative setting? How many caregivers are needed to perform this task safely?
3. In the preoperative area, the caregivers are required to catheterize Mr. H. He has a very large abdominal pannus, obstructing access to the catheterization site. The caregiver will need someone to lift and support the pannus, which weighs approximately 80 lbs. What type of assistance should the caregiver have?
4. At the end of the second day, it was determined that Mr. H could sit in a recliner chair but did not have the strength to transfer. The ceiling lift and sling were identified to fit during the pre-op patient-handling session. Mr. H is experiencing pain and weakness and cannot assist in rolling side to side. What equipment and how many caregivers will be needed to perform this task safely?
5. Mr. H's daily dressing changes on his heel require that his leg be lifted while the bandages are removed and replaced. Prior to surgery, he could assist by lifting his leg for short intervals during the dressing change. After surgery, he is unable to lift his leg. Which method should the caregiver use to lift his leg during the dressing change, and how many caregivers are needed?

Post-Test Questions

3-1. During repositioning of the bariatric patient, the caregiver must consider:
   a. The patient's weight
   b. The size of the bed
   c. The patient's respiratory status
   d. The patient's ability to assist
   e. All of the above
3-2. Bariatric algorithms provide information on which of the following?
   a. The amount of floor space needed to perform the task
   b. The space required in the bed
   c. The number of caregivers required to assist
   d. The patient's medical comorbidities and their relationship to repositioning.
3-3. The bariatric patient may be more sensitive to comments and practices of caregivers that impact the patient's dignity. Which of the following might be disrespectful to the patient?
   a. Ensuring that there are four people available to assist with a bed boost for a 400-lb patient
   b. Posting a sign at the patient's bedside, indicating that because of patient's size, extra precautions are necessary
   c. Labeling equipment as extra capacity (EC) with weight designation
   d. Asking the patient if he or she would like to consult with the dietician

3-4. Mr. Johnson weighs 410 lbs. He cannot assist in turning from side to side or moving himself up in bed. However, he is cooperative. He has slipped down in bed and needs to be repositioned up and turned on his left side. The nurse should do the following:

   a. Using four caregivers, manually reposition the patient up in bed with draw sheet.

   b. Using two–three caregivers, reposition patient up in bed and onto his side using bariatric ceiling-mounted patient lift with supine sling.

   c. Using two caregivers, reposition the patient up in bed using a floor-based patient lift.

   d. Using three caregivers, reposition the patient up in bed using FRDs.

Additional Reading

Acknage, J. (March, 2004). Bariatric products help hospital source growing market. *Healthcare Purchasing News.* Retrieved March 30, 2008, from www.hpnonline.com

Baptiste, A., Boda, S., Nelson, A., Lloyd, J., & Lee, W. (2006). Friction reducing devices for lateral patient transfers: A clinical evaluation. *AAOHN Journal, 54*(4), 173–180.

Davidson, J., & Callery, C. (2001). Care of the obesity surgery patient requiring intermediate level or intensive care. *Obesity Surgery, 11*(1), 93–97.

Department of Veterans Affairs (VHA) VISN 8 Patient Safety Center of Inquiry. (2006). *Safe patient handling and movement algorithms.* Retrieved March 2, 2008, from http://www.visn8.med.va.gov/patientsafetycenter/safePtHandling/default.asp

Hahler, B. (2002). Morbid obesity: A nursing care challenge. *Medsurg Nursing, 11*(2), 85–90.

Klein, M. (n.d.). Treating obese patients the right way. *Healthcare Purchasing News.* Retrieved on March 30, 2008, from www.hypnonline.com

Marras, W. S., Davis, K. G., Kirking, B. C., Bertsche, P. K. (1999). A comprehensive analysis of low back disorder risk and spinal loading during the transferring and repositioning of patients using different techniques. *Ergonomics, 42*, 904–926.

McGill, S., & Kavcic, N. (2005). Transfer of the horizontal patient: The effect of a friction reducing assistive device on low back mechanics. *Ergonomics, 48*(8), 915–929.

Muir, M. (2005). The bariatric resident. In *Guideline for Architects and Facility Space Planners, 2nd Edition.* Eslov, Sweden, ARJO AB.

Muir, M., Archer-Heese, G., McLean, D., Bodnar, S., & Rock, B. L. (2007). A case study of a bariatric patient in the MICU: Problems and solutions. *Critical Care Journal of North America, 19*(2), 223–240.

Muir, M. (2004). Morbidly obese patient care and staff safety issues. Novations Conference May 25, 2004.

Proteau, R.-A., & Marchand, D. (n.d.) Impact of bedding surfaces on effort required to reposition clients to the head of the bed. Quebec, Canada: ASSTSAS.

Vieira, E. R. (n.d.). Risk assessment of bariatric patient transfers from bed to wheelchair. Edmonton, Alberta Canada: University of Alberta.

Villeneuve, J., Poulind, P., & Bertrand, G. (2007). Des amenagements adaptes pour la clientele obese. *Objectiv Prevention ASSTSAS, 30*(5), 22–25.

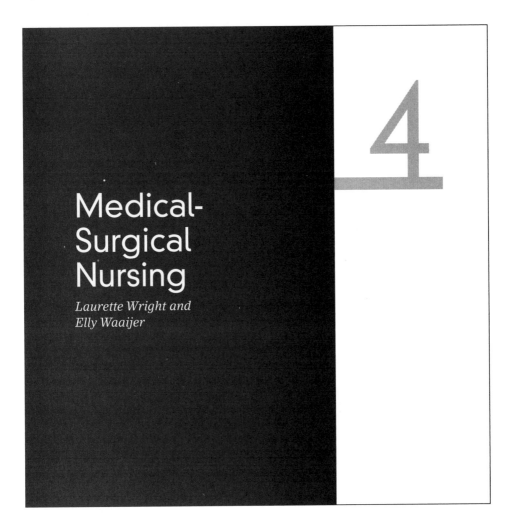

4

Medical-Surgical Nursing

*Laurette Wright and
Elly Waaijer*

Description of Setting

The practice of medical-surgical nursing involves understanding the complexity of clinical and surgical conditions affecting the adult population. These conditions range from diabetes and cardiovascular disease to multiple organ dysfunction (Lewis, Heitkemper & Dirksen, 2007). Patients are adults whose body weights far exceed the 35-lb limit for manual handling (Waters, 2007), necessitating that caregivers use patient handling devices for all high-risk tasks.

Unique Challenges to Providing Safe Patient Handling in this Setting

The biggest challenge in safe patient handling on general medical or surgical units is that the patient's condition fluctuates over the course of a day (e.g., due to medications or fatigue), as well as over the course of the hospital stay.

Medical-surgical patients present themselves with a wide range of mobility levels that may change within hours of being admitted. For example, the patient may be ambulatory upon admission, bedridden following a surgical procedure, and then independent upon discharge. This dynamic change in the patient's physical condition provides unique problem-solving challenges for the caregiver, who is responsible for providing high-quality care in a manner that is safe for the patient, safe for the caregiver, and consistent with the patient's therapy.

High-Risk Tasks

The high-risk tasks associated with medical-surgical units include the following:

- Tasks involving hospital beds
- Placing and removing bedpan
- Toileting using sit-to-stand patient lift
- Toileting using floor-based or ceiling-mounted patient lift
- Application of compression stockings
- Dressing/wound care of the extremities
- Postmortem care: transfer to morgue cart using friction-reducing devices (FRDs)
- Postmortem care: transfer to morgue cart using floor-based or ceiling-mounted patient lift

Objectives

1. Describe the unique risks associated with safe patient handling in medical-surgical patient populations.
2. Identify three high-risk patient-handling tasks on medical/surgical units.
3. For each high-risk patient-handling task, delineate the number of caregivers and types of equipment needed, and tips for performing the task safely.

Pre-Test Questions

4-1. What approach to toileting best promotes safe patient handling?
   a. Regardless of the patient's condition, promote use of a bedpan or urinal so that you do not have to transfer the patient.
   b. Use of a patient a floor-based lift or ceiling-mounted lift with hygiene sling to transfer a physically dependent patient to a toilet.
   c. Manually lift a patient who is ambulatory but confused and agitated, using soothing tone of voice to escort to the toilet.
   d. Always have two or three caregivers present when completing toileting tasks.

4-2. When providing care to a physically dependent patient, what is the best approach for placing/removing a bedpan?
   a. Use a patient lift to allow you to safely insert or remove the bedpan.
   b. Ask the patient to support the movement as much as possible.
   c. Place the patient in a comfortable position with the head of the bed raised to a comfortable level and at elbow level.
   d. All of the above.

4-3. What is the safest approach for applying and removing compression stockings?
   a. Let the patient perform task if capable.
   b. This is not a high-risk task, and there is no need for use of an assistive device.
   c. Apply the stocking from the side of the bed rather than the foot.
   d. Use assistive device for application of compression stockings.

4-4. When performing wound care and a dressing to the lower extremity while the patient is in bed, the following safe patient-handling and movement strategy should be used:
   a. Use limb-lifting sling for entire procedure.
   b. Have another health care worker hold limb.
   c. Transfer patient out of bed first.
   d. Use limb-lifting sling for removal of old dressing only.

4-5. While performing postmortem care it is necessary to keep the following in mind:
   a. There are no algorithms for postmortem care.
   b. The body can be easily moved without the use of assistive devices.
   c. Ceiling-mounted patient lift and repositioning sling can be used while performing care.
   d. None of the above.

General Directions for All Tasks

1. Complete *Assessment Criteria and Care Plan* for patient. Key assessment factors include physical ability to assist, ability to follow instructions, and cooperation. *Note: Weight and height may trigger use of bariatric algorithms.*
2. Review the algorithm for the high-risk patient-handling task to be performed and determine the number of caregivers, types of equipment, and techniques for performing each high-risk patient-handling task safely. If no algorithm exists, use the techniques described in this book to guide practice.
3. Check the weight capacity of the equipment to be sure it is safe to handle the patient's weight.
4. Remove obstacles to performing the patient-handling tasks. Obstacles include too little room to maneuver the equipment, equipment stored on the floor posing a stumbling hazard, or inability to perform the activity without threats to patient dignity (e.g., lack of privacy). You may need to remove chairs or bed tables, separate beds, move floor-based equipment, and ask visitors to leave.

5. Make sure selected equipment is in good working order. If the equipment is battery operated, check that the battery is charged. Verify that the appropriate slings and attachments are available. Review safe operation of the equipment, including location of emergency buttons or manual controls for the event of a power failure.
6. Ensure sufficient caregivers are available to help, as specified in the algorithm.
7. Make sure beds are adjusted to caregiver's waist/elbow height before performing bed-related patient-handling tasks.
8. Explain the procedure to the patient and assisting caregivers.
9. Wear gloves according to proper infection-control practices and facility policies.

Placing and Removing Bedpan

Description of Task and Associated Risks

While placing and removing a bedpan, the caregiver provides assistance to the patient as needed. Using a bedpan requires some coordination and cooperation on the part of the patient. Risks to the caregiver include lifting heavy loads, awkward postures, and frequency; this is a common task. Potential risks to the patient include skin shearing and tissue damage from sitting on a bedpan for a prolonged period.

Patient Abilities

- Partially able to assist in bed positioning
- Cooperative

Resources Required

- Friction-reducing device (FRD) or repositioning sling with lift to position patient on side if patient unable to do this independently
- One caregiver (Additional caregiver may be needed if FRD is used.)
- Supplies needed for bedpan use

Technique 4-1

1. Follow *General Directions for All Tasks.*
2. If a patient is bedridden but still able to do all the moving him/herself, it is quite easy to place and remove a bedpan. As always, it is important to encourage the patient to do as much as possible for him/herself.
3. If patient assistance is needed, consider using an FRD or repositioning sling to turn the patient to the side to insert or remove bedpan.
4. Roll the patient to a supine position to insert the bedpan and position for comfort with the head raised and legs slightly spread.

4.1

Positioning the
patient on
his/her side

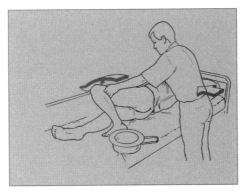

4.2

Sliding the bedpan
under the patient

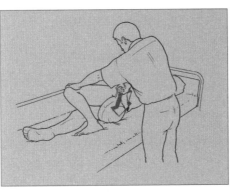

4.3

Positioning
the patient on
the bedpan

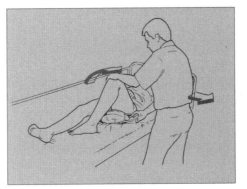

4.4

The patient properly
positioned on the
bedpan

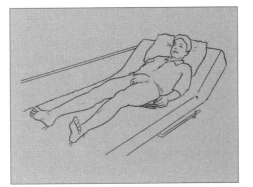

4.5

Removing
the bedpan
(Knibbe, 2008)

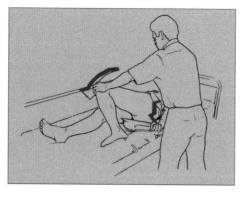

Application of Compression Stockings

Description of Task and Associated Risks

Compression stockings (also known as anti-embolism stockings) are widely used for the prevention of deep vein thrombosis (DVT) or for the management of long-term venous insufficiency. Unfortunately, the application and removal of the correctly sized stockings is considered a high-risk task because of the high force and gripping on the caregiver's hands and the excessive weight lifted and held in awkward positions when applying or removing the stocking. The patient is at risk for skin shearing (Knibbe & Knibbe, 2008).

View Video 4.1: Compression Stockings: Application and Removal.

Patient Abilities

■ Independent application
  1. Upper-extremity strength and hand function
  2. Trunk support and ability to reach feet
■ Partial assistance
  1. Limited extremity strength and hand function
  2. Limited trunk support and ability to reach
■ Total assistance
  1. Insufficient strength and hand function
  2. Insufficient trunk support and ability to reach

Resources Required

■ Compression stockings (correct size for patient)
■ Compression stocking applicator
■ One caregiver (either performs task or coaches patient to perform task)

Technique 4-2

1. Follow the *General Directions for All Tasks.*
2. Prepare to apply/remove compression stockings.
3. Check whether or not the patient's compression stocking has an open toe.

Helpful Hint

Have household gloves available, preferably the ones with uneven surface on the fingers. This enables the patient to have more grip on the stockings to roll them over his/her legs.

4. Select the right compression stocking applicator (open versus closed toe), making sure to select the correct size.
5. Select the right compression stocking take-off aid (same for open and closed toe)
6. Option 1: Patient performs task.
   a. If patient is able to perform task independently, provide a solid chair that allows patient's feet to reach the floor.
   Option 2: Patient performs task with caregiver assistance (seated position).
   a. Provide a solid chair for the patient that allows patient's feet to reach the floor.
   b. Caregiver should use height-adjustable, working chair to minimize stress on the back while performing this task. Ask the patient to put his/her leg on your knees. This enables the caregiver to work in a less stressful posture. If needed, first place a small cushion or towel on your knees.
   Option 3: Caregiver performs task (patient lying in bed).
   a. Patient should be in bed, with head of the bed slightly elevated. Position feet at the end of the bed.
   b. Using a compression-stocking applicator (open vs. closed toe) with the correct size of stocking, the caregiver should stand at the foot of the bed (caregiver's face towards foot end) to avoid awkward postures, twisting, and turning.
7. Follow these steps to apply compression stockings:
   a. Bring the compression stocking applicator over the foot
   b. Bring the stocking over the heel while rubbing the stocking over the smooth surface of the aid.
   c. If the stocking is over the heel, take away the aid through the open toe end. If it is a closed stocking, pull on the right loop to get the aid out of the stocking.
   d. Rub the stocking over the leg or ask the patient to do the last part him/herself.
   e. Make a visual check to ensure the stocking fits well around the leg.

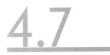

4.6

Anti-embolism stocking

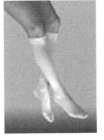

4.7

Anti-embolism stocking (thigh high)

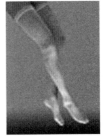

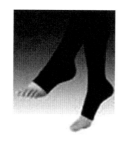

4.8

Anti-embolism
stocking (open toe)

8. Follow these steps to remove compression stockings:
    a. Bring the take-off aid around the patient's foot
    b. Rub the stocking over the leg
    c. While reaching the foot rub the stocking over the smooth surface of the take-off aid till the stocking comes over the heel and complete foot

Toileting Using Stand-Assist Lift

Depending on the patient's ability, the task of toileting can be very complex, particularly as you take into consideration the patient's room environment (e.g., entry threshold to private bathroom) in addition to the patient's mobility level. Toileting includes not only the ability to get the patient on and off a commode (e.g., bedside commode and stationary commode in private bath), but also the changing of incontinence pads that are used for urine, bowel motions, and female discharge (menses) (NBPA & Royal College of Nursing, 1997). The purpose of this section is to highlight the task of toileting using a stand-assist lift. The advantage of a stand-assist lift is that the sling typically fits around the patient's back above the waistline and is out of the way of toileting tasks.

View Video 4.2: Toileting Using
Stand-Assist Lift

Description of Risks

Risk factors for the caregiver include sustained awkward postures, reaching, lifting heavy loads, and twisting.

Patient Abilities

- Limited trunk support/balance deficits
- Ability to bear full weight on extremities
- Cooperative

Resources Required

- Stand-assist lift and appropriate sling

Technique 4-3

1. Ensure floor clearance for transferring patient from bed to commode.
2. Raise patient's bed to appropriate height for caregiver.
3. Insert sling in accordance with manufacturer's guidelines.

4. Attach sling to lift's hanger bar.
5. Transport patient to the toilet area.
6. Transfer patient from bed to commode. (Remove or adjust patient's clothing prior to placement onto commode surface, if necessary.)
7. Assist with perineal care following completion of toileting.
8. Return patient to bed.
9. Remove the sling and the mechanical lift.

Toileting Using Floor-Based or Ceiling-Mounted Patient Lift

Depending on the patient's ability, the task of toileting can be very complex, particularly as you take into consideration the patient's room environment (e.g., entry threshold to private bathroom) in addition to the patient's mobility level. Toileting includes not only the ability to get the patient on and off a commode (e.g., bedside commode and stationary commode in private bath), but also the changing of incontinence pads that are used for urine, bowel motions, and female discharge (menses) (NBPA & Royal College of Nursing, 1997). The purpose of this section is to highlight the tasks of using a floor-based patient lift in combination with specialty slings designed specifically for toileting. These slings allow for the adjustment of the patient's clothing.

> View Video 4.3: Toileting Using Floor-Based or Ceiling-Mounted Patient Lift

NOTE: Most toileting slings require that the patient generally have good trunk support because the design of the sling fits around the patient's chest and does not extend upward to support the head and neck area. Therefore, the less muscle tone the patient has, the less likely he or she is suitable for this type of sling. The leg sections usually allow for the patient's hips and buttocks to be clear for easy access by the health care provider to provide perineal care and/or clothing adjustment.

NOTE: If a toileting sling is not available, consider using a sling that can be easily wiped with approved hospital disinfectant OR use a patient-specific/disposable standard sling that can be discarded if it becomes heavily soiled with body fluids such as feces, blood, or urine.

Description of Risks

Risk factors for the caregiver include sustained awkward postures, reaching, lifting heavy loads, and twisting.

Patient Abilities

- Limited trunk support or balance deficit
- Limited ability to bear weight
- Possibly uncooperative

Resources Required

- Sling (toileting style preferred)
- Floor-based or ceiling-mounted patient lift
- Bedside commode (if applicable)

Technique 4-4

1. Ensure sufficient floor clearance for transferring patient from bed to commode.
2. Raise patient's bed to appropriate height for caregiver.
3. Insert sling in accordance with manufacturer's guidelines.
4. Attach sling to lift's hanger bar.
5. Transfer patient from bed to commode. (Remove or adjust patient's clothing prior to placement onto commode surface, if necessary.)
6. Assist with perineal care following completion of toileting.
7. Return patient to bed.
8. Remove the sling and the mechanical lift.

Tasks Involving Hospital Beds

Description of Task and Associated Risks

Beds are central to hospital life. A good hospital bed provides a safe environment for the patient and is easy and intuitive for both patients and caregivers to use. It provides clinical benefits for the patient, as well as a comfortable support surface. Additionally, it contributes to improved efficiency and helps to reduce the staff's risk of moving and handling injuries. The patient-handling issues surrounding the hospital bed remain an area of great importance. A good hospital bed must be designed to minimize such risks, and it should enable staff to move patients with safety, dignity, and ease.

Some of the common moving and handling tasks performed in and around a hospital bed include these:

- Transferring on/off bedpan
- Assisting into/out of bed
- Feeding
- Turning and repositioning to prevent pressure ulcers
- Bathing
- (Un)dressing
- Performing treatments, such as dressings
- Assisting/performing portable check xrays.

The benefits of electric profiling beds (beds with special features built in to facilitate adjustments to position the patient) are now very well recognized. Four-section profiling beds place and maintain patients in a much better sitting position than flat-base and two-section beds. Placing patients in an upright position actively benefits all major body systems while providing important psychological benefits. If the bed is used in a proper way, it also can support the movement of bringing the patient from a supine position to a sitting position on the edge of the bed. If upright positioning is combined with mobilization, the benefits are further increased, resulting in faster recovery from illness and improved clinical outcomes.

A number of studies have shown that four-section, electric profiling beds offer advantages when combined with good-quality, pressure-reducing and pressure-relieving mattresses. These advantages include a reduction in pressure-ulcer incidence, an increase in patient independence, a reduction in the amount of nursing time taken up with patient-handling tasks such as those listed above and a reduction in moving and handling injuries to staff (Caboor et al., 2000).

Bed transfers were described in chapter 2 and will not be repeated here. Rather, we focus on reducing the need to reposition the patient in the bed through the use of profiling beds. Patients slide down in bed because they are in sitting positions, supported by pillows or by a raised head of the bed. This position causes a patient to slide 10–15 cm downward in the bed, causing discomfort and requiring repositioning. To solve this problem in an optimal way, some beds automatically raise the leg rest before the backrest comes to a sitting position. By using a four-section profiled bed in the right manner, the caregiver can reduce the need to perform the high-risk task of repositioning patients in bed.

Patient Ability

■ Unable to assist or partially able to assist

Resources Required

■ A four-section bed is the optimum solution for reducing the number of transfers in bed. If the bed has fewer sections, adapt the technique to the functionality of the bed.

Technique 4-5

1. Follow *General Directions for All Tasks*.
2. Read the operating instructions for the bed.
3. Provide a comprehensive operating instruction of the bed to those patients who can operate the bed themselves.
4. If the bed does not automatically raise the leg rest before the backrest is raised, do so manually while bringing the patient to a sitting position.
5. If the patient wants to lie down, reverse the order. First bring the back rest down, then the leg rest.
6. If the bed does not have automated sections and therefore requires the use of support pillows, it is advisable to give some extra support under the upper legs before placing pillows behind the patient's back. This is not ideal but sometimes is seen in practice.

Dressing/Wound Care of the Extremities

Description of Task and Associated Risks

Caregivers provide various types of wound care to patients, ranging from debridement of a burn area to the application of wet gauze material that has been soaked with antimicrobial or coated with topical creams. It is the frequency and duration of these dressing changes, combined with the awkward postures of the patient or caregiver, that often result in unsatisfactory working postures. Therefore, this routine task is high risk.

When the caregiver takes on the task of lifting a portion of the patient's body weight, such as holding the arm or leg, he/she risks *static overload* (keeping the body in the same position for prolonged period of time). It is this static overload, combined with the amount of force required to lift and hold the limb, that contributes to caregiver musculoskeletal injuries such as shoulder, upper back, and arm injuries. Studies suggest that one leg equals 30% of a person's total body weight and can easily exceed the 35-lb weight limit for manual handling (Waters, 2007).

> View Video 4.4: Dressing/
> Wound Care of the Extremities

Therefore, to minimize this type of overload during dressing changes of a patient's extremities, take the following precautions:

- Use adjustable equipment whenever possible—bed, chairs, and bedside trays.
- Use leg- or arm-lifting equipment to support the patient's body part and allow easier access by caregiver while performing wound care.

Patient Abilities

- Any status that requires external assistance to hold limb in stationary position

Resources Required

- Ceiling-mounted patient lift or floor-based patient lift (with loop attachments)
- Limb sling
- One–two caregivers (depending on patient's weight or arm/leg girth)
- Wound-care supplies

Technique 4-6

1. Get limb sling and ensure appropriate lift is available in patient's room.
2. Gather wound-care supplies or kit.
3. Elevate patient's bed to comfortable height using adjustable bed controls.
4. Gently position the limb sling underneath the patient's leg/arm while keeping one hand between the sling fabric and the patient's skin. Ensure even amounts of sling are on each side.

   NOTE: Do not place limb sling directly underneath joints such as the wrist, elbow, or knee

Helpful Hint

You may insert a friction-reducing device (FRD) underneath the patient's limb prior to inserting the limb sling to minimize friction of the sling directly against the patient's skin. Remove the FRD once the limb sling is positioned and BEFORE attachment of the sling to the mechanical lift.

5. Use the lift's controls to lower the spreader bar toward the limb-sling attachments.
6. Attach the loops of the limb sling. Ensure that the attachments are secured to the hanger bar.
7. Operate the lift's controls to raise the patient's limb to desired height, avoiding hyperextension of the extremity.
8. Perform wound care.
9. Use the lift's controls to lower the patient's leg/arm to the bed.
10. Remove the limb sling.

Postmortem Care: Transfer to Morgue Cart Using FRDs

Description of Task and Associated Risks

Postmortem care is the care provided to a patient immediately after death. It is important to maintain patient dignity and proper patient body alignment, with minimal occurrence of skin damage or discoloration. Rigor mortis, the stiffening of the deceased muscles, will begin to occur within 2 to 4 hours after death, which may cause difficulty in positioning the body (Beattie, 2006; Harvey, 2001). Risks associated with postmortem care include lifting heavy weight, pushing/pulling forces, sustained awkward positioning, excessive reach, and long duration of task. Because the task is of long duration, it is important to have the bed at the correct height (elbow/waist level). Additionally, risk is associated with positioning the patient while preparing the body, as well as during patient transfer from bed to morgue cart.

> View Video 4.5: Transfer to Morgue Cart Using Friction Reducing Devices

Patient Abilities

- Not applicable

Resources Required

- FRD
- Stretcher or morgue cart
- Two–three caregivers, depending on patient's weight
- Postmortem supplies, typically provided in a kit

Technique 4-7

1. Follow *General Directions for All Tasks*.
2. Perform postmortem care with the patient's bed in a semi-Fowler position. (Use FRD or patient lift to assist with positioning body for access needed to complete care.)
3. Adjust patient's bed to supine position to prepare for patient transfer. Arrange bed and stretcher/morgue cart so that morgue cart is slightly lower than the bed and all casters are locked on both bed and cart.

Helpful Hint

Place postmortem bag on top of FRD and insert both items together. This allows for easier adjustment of patient's body inside of the bag.

4. Position patient on side using log-roll technique and insert FRD under patient, using more than one if needed to fit the length and width of the body surface in contact with the mattress.

Helpful Hint

If FRDs have handles, use gait belt, towel, or pillowcases and insert through handles to create "extenders." This technique will reduce amount of upper-back flexion and static load of the caregiver during the transfer.

5. Using two or three caregivers, grasp the side edges of the FRD or use the handles (if available), and, in a coordinated fashion, laterally transfer patient to stretcher/morgue cart.
6. Remove FRD.

Postmortem Care: Transfer to Morgue Cart Using Floor-Based or Ceiling-Mounted Patient Lift

Description of Task and Associated Risks

Postmortem care is the care provided to a patient immediately after death. It is important to maintain patient dignity and proper patient body alignment, with minimal occurrence of skin damage or discoloration. Rigor mortis, the stiffening of the deceased muscles, will begin to occur within 2 to 4 hours after death, which may cause difficulty in positioning the body (Beattie, 2006; Harvey, 2001). Risks associated with postmortem care include lifting heavy weight, pushing/pulling forces, sustained awkward positioning, excessive reach, and long duration of task. Because the task is of long duration, it is important to have the bed at the correct height (elbow/waist level). Additionally, risk is associated with positioning the patient while preparing the body, as well as during patient transfer from bed to morgue cart.

View Video 4.6: Transfer to Morgue Cart Using Floor-Based or Ceiling-Mounted Patient Lift

Patient Abilities

- Not applicable

Resources Required

- Floor-based patient lift (with supine sling, not always available with this device) or ceiling-mounted patient lift (with supine sling)
- Stretcher or morgue cart
- Two caregivers when using floor-based or ceiling-mounted patient lift
- Postmortem supplies, typically provided in a kit

Technique 4-8

1. Follow *General Directions for All Tasks*.
2. Perform postmortem care with the patient's bed in a semi-Fowler position. (Use FRD or patient lift to assist with positioning body for access needed to complete care.)
3. Adjust patient's bed to supine position to prepare for patient transfer. Arrange bed and stretcher/morgue cart so that morgue cart is slightly lower than the bed and all casters are locked on both bed and cart.
4. Position the patient's body onto the supine sling by rolling the body toward one caregiver, then folding the sling in half, placing it behind the back, and rolling the body to the other side to pull the sling through.
5. Connect the sling to the patient lift.
6. Move the body toward the center of the morgue stretcher/cart. Lower the spreader bar until patient's body is securely placed on the stretcher.
7. Remove sling straps from all sides of the patient.

Case Study 4-1

Sarah Johnston is 55-year-old woman who weighs 125 lbs. She has been receiving chemotherapy for ovarian cancer on an outpatient basis. She completed her third treatment 5 days ago and has been experiencing severe nausea and vomiting, although she has been taking antiemetic medication at home to help alleviate those symptoms. Upon admission to the medical-surgical unit, Ms. Johnston complained of periodic episodes of lethargy, weakness, and dizziness. At times she is able to position herself to the side of the bed and assist the nurse with stand pivot in using the bedside commode, without the use of any mechanical-assistance devices. During the evening hours, Ms. Johnston frequently experiences generalized weakness, which prevents her from assisting the staff in getting her to a bedside commode or to her private bathroom facility.

Discussion Questions

1. Based on her clinical manifestations, what is the most preferable technique(s) for promoting bowel/bladder control for Ms. Johnston?
2. What additional assessment factors should be considered in determining the correct mechanical lift or assistive device?

Case Study 4-2

Mr. Alexander is a 62-year-old man who weighs 190 lbs. He has been admitted to the unit with compromised circulation of the right lower leg and necrotic areas on his right foot. He is a diabetic and has not been consistent in taking his insulin; therefore, his blood glucose has not been well controlled. He is alert and has good upper-body strength; however, he complains of numbness and tingling in his right leg. He has experienced a high-grade temperature of 101° within the past 48 hours. Mr. Alexander refuses to use the bedpan and wants to ambulate to the restroom with the assistance of two nurses. Mr. Alexander's physician has ordered isolation precautions in addition to wound-dressing changes to his right foot three times per day.

Discussion Questions:

1. Based on the assessment data presented, what are your plans and interventions for conducting wound care?
2. Based on the assessment data presented, what are your plans and interventions for conducting bowel and bladder management?

Post-Test Questions

4-1. What approach to toileting best promotes safe patient handling?
   a. Regardless of the patient's condition, promote use of a bedpan or urinal so that you do not have to transfer the patient.
   b. Use of a patient a floor-based lift or ceiling-mounted lift with hygiene sling to transfer a physically dependent patient to a toilet.
   c. Manually lift a patient who is ambulatory but confused and agitated, using soothing tone of voice to escort to the toilet.
   d. Always have two or three caregivers present when completing toileting tasks.
4-2. When providing care to a physically dependent patient, what is the best approach for placing/removing a bedpan?
   a. Use a patient lift to allow you to safely insert or remove the bedpan.
   b. Ask the patient to support the movement as much as possible.
   c. Place the patient in a comfortable position with the head of the bed raised to a comfortable level and at elbow level.
   d. All of the above.
4-3. What is the safest approach for applying and removing compression stockings?
   a. Let the patient perform task if capable.
   b. This is not a high-risk task, and there is no need for use of an assistive device.
   c. Apply the stocking from the side of the bed rather than the foot.
   d. Use assistive device for application of compression stockings.

4-4. When performing wound care and a dressing to the lower extremity while the patient is in bed, the following safe patient-handling and movement strategy should be used:

    a. Use limb-lifting sling for entire procedure.

    b. Have another health care worker hold limb.

    c. Transfer patient out of bed first.

    d. Use limb-lifting sling for removal of old dressing only.

4-5. While performing postmortem care it is necessary to keep the following in mind:

    a. There are no algorithms for postmortem care.

    b. The body can be easily moved without the use of assistive devices.

    c. Ceiling-mounted lift and repositioning sling can be used while performing care.

    d. None of the above are correct.

References

Beattie, S. (October 2006) Post-mortem care. RNweb. Retrieved April 6, 2008, from http://rn.modernmedicine.com/rnweb/Acute+Care+Focus/Post-mortem-care/ArticleStandard/Article/detail/375514

Caboor, D., Verlinden, M., Zinzen, E., Van Roy, P., Van Riel, M., & Clarys, J. (2000). Implications of an adjustable bed height during standard nursing tasks on spinal motion, perceived exertion and muscular activity. *Ergonomics, 43*(10), 1771–1780.

Harvey, Jeff. (2001). Debunking myths about postmortem care. *Nursing, 31*(7), 44–45. Retrieved on April 6, 2008, from http://findarticles. com/p/articles/mi_qa3689/is_200107/ai_n9002202/pg_2

Knibbe, J. J., Van Panhuys, W., Van Vught, W., Hooghiemstra, F., & Waaijer, E. M. (2008). Handbook of transfers. UK: Diligent.

Lewis, S., Heitkemper, M. M., & Dirksen, S. R. (2007). *Medical-surgical nursing: Assessment and management of clinical problems.* Philadelphia, PA: Mosby Elsevier.

NBPA (National Back Pain Association) & Royal College of Nursing. (1997). *The guide to the handling of patients: Introducing a safer handling policy* (4th ed.). Teddington, Middlesex, United Kingdom: National Back Pain Association.

Waters, T. R. (2007). When is it safe to manually lift a patient? The Revised NIOSH Lifting Equation provides support for recommended weight limits. *American Journal of Nursing, 107*(8), 53–58.

Additional Reading

ARJO AB. (2005). *ARJO guidebook for architects and planners.* Eslov, Sweden: ARJO AB.

Baptiste, A. (2007). Technology solutions for high-risk tasks in critical care. *Critical Care Nursing Clinics of North America, 19*(2), 177–186.

Birtles, M., & Williams, S. (2004). An ergonomic evaluation of hospital backrests. *The Column, 16*(2), 18–20.

Chaffin, D. B., Andersson, G. B. J., & Martin B. J. (1999). *Occupational biomechanics* (3rd ed.). New York: Wiley & Sons.

Demain, S., Gore, S., & McLellan, D. L. (2000). The use of leg lifting equipment. *Nursing Standard, 14,* (39), 41–43.

Jensen, R. K. (1989). Changes in segment inertia proportions between four and twenty years. *Journal of Biomechanics, 22*(6–7), 529–536.

Keogh, A., & Dealey, C. (2001). Profiling beds versus standard beds: Effects on pressure ulcer incidence outcomes. *Journal of Wound Care, 2,* 15–19.

Knibbe, J. J., & Knibbe, N. E. (2006). *Monitoring the effects of ergonomic covenants for workers in Dutch healthcare.* LOCOmotion, I.E.A. congress Maastricht NL.

Mital, A., Nicholson, A. S., & Ayoub, M. M. (1997). *A guide to manual materials handling.* London: Taylor & Francis.

Murphy, D., Charles, S., Monnington, S., & Powell, R. (2005). The impact of profiling beds on manual handling risk and patient experience. *The Column, 17*(4), 18–21.

Nelson, A. L. (Ed.). (2006). *Safe patient handling and movement: A practical guide for health care professionals.* New York: Springer.

NICE CG46 Venous Thromboembolism. (2007). Available at www.nice.org.uk.

Robotham, R. (2003). Risk: The cost of not being prepared. *The Column, 15*(3), 12–15.

Tarling, C., & Burns, N. (1994). Let the bed take the strain. *Professional Caregiver, 9*, 759–763.

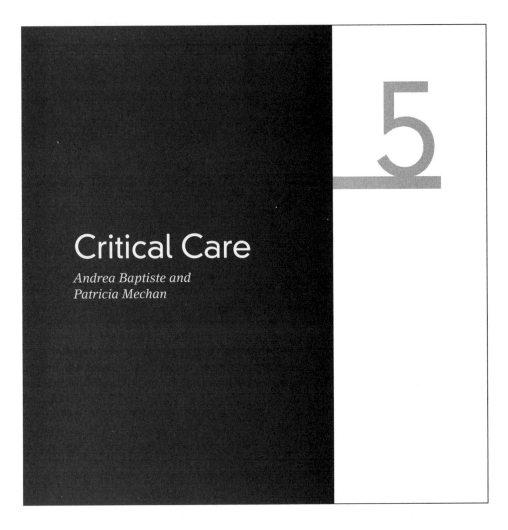

Critical Care

Andrea Baptiste and
Patricia Mechan

Description of Setting

Critical care settings, also known as intensive care units, are often fast paced and unpredictable, which increases the risk of musculoskeletal injuries associated with patient handling. (Waters, Nelson, Proctor, 2007) Patients in critical care are generally physically dependent and may be confused or have difficulty following instructions due to illness/injury, medications, or cognition. The purpose of this chapter is to identify high-risk patient-handling tasks and outline practical solutions applicable to critical care settings.

Unique Challenges to Providing Safe Patient Handling in this Setting

The medical condition of a patient changes rapidly in critical care and often requires the caregiver to frequently assess and reassess functional status and safe patient-handling needs. Critical care environments are typically crowded with equipment and personnel, forcing caregivers into awkward positions. Caregivers must frequently transport patients off the unit (e.g., diagnostic areas, surgery, radiology), increasing risk associated with pushing and pulling occupied beds or stretchers.

High-Risk Tasks

The following high-risk tasks have been identified:

1. Positioning and holding legs for access to perineum
2. Patient transport
3. Positioning for bedside X-ray
4. Positioning for treatments (turning for wound management/dressings, access)

Objectives

1. Describe the unique challenges associated with safe patient handling in critical care.
2. Identify high-risk patient-handling tasks on critical care units.
3. Delineate the number of caregivers, types of equipment, and techniques used for performing each high-risk patient-handling task safely.

Pre-Test Questions

5-1. You are the nurse caring for a female patient who is on a ventilator and in a coma. You will be inserting a Foley catheter. What is the best choice of equipment for this task?
   a. Use a sling that will lift and support limb(s) for procedure.
   b. Have two health care workers hold both legs in position for procedure.
   c. Have one other health care worker hold both legs in position for procedure.
   d. None of the above are correct.
5-2. What patient-care task has the potential for staff injury in critical care?
   a. Repositioning, "boosting up" in bed
   b. Turning patient
   c. Positioning patient for procedures or exams
   d. All of the above
5-3. Sustained holding of a patient's leg has been identified as a high-risk task in critical care. Why is it a physically demanding task?
   a. Because of the weight of the leg
   b. Because of the size of the leg
   c. Because of the awkward posture that the caregiver adopts when holding the leg
   d. Because of all of the above

5-4. Which of the following statements is *not* true?
   a. There are two types of patient-transport devices: detachable and integrated.
   b. Integrated patient-transport devices are those that can attach to a bed, trolley, or cart.
   c. Integrated devices are typically more expensive than detachable devices.
   d. Patient transport devices are a good option because they can reduce the push forces involved in moving beds, carts, or trolleys.

5-5. You are the nurse caring for a patient in the intensive care unit. This patient will be transported to another floor in his bed. He has chest tubes and a ventilator. What is the best method for transferring this patient?
   a. Bed mover to move bed
   b. One health care worker for ventilator
   c. One health care worker for chest tubes
   d. All of the above

General Directions for All Tasks

1. Complete *Assessment Criteria and Care Plan* for patient. Key assessment factors include physical ability to assist, ability to follow instructions, and cooperation. *Note: Weight and height may trigger use of bariatric algorithms.*
2. Review the algorithm for the high-risk patient-handling task to be performed and determine the number of caregivers, types of equipment, and techniques for performing each high-risk patient-handling task safely. If no algorithm exists, use the techniques described in this book to guide practice.
3. Check the weight capacity of the equipment to be sure it can accommodate the patient's weight.
4. Remove obstacles to performing the patient-handling tasks. Obstacles include too little room to maneuver the equipment, equipment stored on the floor posing a stumbling hazard, or inability to perform the activity without threats to patient dignity (e.g., lack of privacy). You may need to remove chairs or bed tables, separate beds, move floor-based equipment, and ask visitors to leave.
5. Make sure selected equipment is in good working order. If the equipment is battery operated, check that the battery is charged. Verify that the appropriate slings and attachments are available. Review safe operation of the equipment, including location of emergency buttons or manual controls in the event of a power failure.
6. Ensure sufficient caregivers are available to help, as specified in the algorithm.
7. Make sure beds are adjusted to caregiver's waist/elbow height before performing bed-related patient-handling tasks.
8. Explain the procedure to the patient and assisting caregivers.
9. Wear gloves according to proper infection-control practices and facility policies.

Positioning and Holding Legs for Access to Perineum

Description of Task and Associated Risks

In critical care, patients usually have mobility limitations and are functionally dependent. Nurses often require adequate access to the perineum for care, including, but not limited to, catheter insertion, hygiene tasks, and skin and wound treatments. This becomes a handling and lifting risk when (1) patients are unable to move and sustain their legs in a position to allow the nurse sufficient visual and physical access, and (2) the task is performed on patients with large abdomen and limbs with excess tissue that can obscure visual and physical access. (Refer to Chapter 3, Bariatrics.) For nonbariatric patients, use the 35- lb, recommended maximum limit for lifting patients and body parts (Waters, 2007). Risks to caregivers include awkward postures, tasks of long duration, and reaching.

Patient Abilities

- ■ Able to assist in the placement of the sling and its leg straps

Resources Required

- ■ Sling with divided leg straps
- ■ Lifting device, such as a ceiling-mounted or floor-based patient lift with a hanger/spreader bar that can be centered over the patient in the bed
- ■ One caregiver (two caregivers needed if the patient is uncooperative)

Technique 5-1

1. Follow *General Instructions for all Tasks.*
2. Place patient in supine position with the head of bed at height comfortable for the patient.
3. Place the universal sling beneath the patient, with each divided leg strap beneath its corresponding limb.
4. Attach the leg straps via their connecting loops to the lift's hanger bar.
5. Raise the height of the hanger bar, while watching the position of the patient, until desired position of limbs and access are achieved.
6. Reverse steps to remove sling from beneath patient.

5.1

Positioning and
holding legs for
access to perineum—
starting position

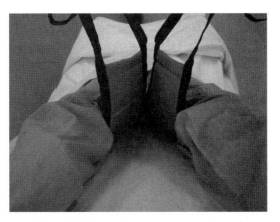

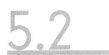

5.2

Positioning and
holding legs for
access to perineum—
ending position

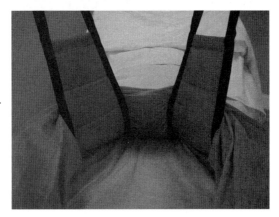

Patient Transport

Description of Task and Associated Risks

Patient transport has been identified as a high-risk task due to the high forces required to move heavy beds occupied with a patient. The average weight of a bed in critical care is approximately 600–700 lbs, and the combined weight of bed and patient can easily approach 1,000 lbs.

In addition to the weight of the patient and bed/stretcher, the difficulty of the task is compounded by added medical devices (e.g., intra-aortic balloon pumps, intravenous pumps, and portable ventilators). Additionally, nurses are expected to monitor the patient while performing this task or manually ventilating the patient and walking/pushing. Because the task requires two or more persons for safety, at least one person is walking backwards. Pushing is preferable over pulling, but neither is considered safe when performed manually.

> View Video 5.1: Patient Transport with Power Drive Bed

Patient Abilities

- Not applicable; patients in critical care do not move out of unit unassisted

Resources Required

There are two types of devices that can facilitate easier patient transport. The first is the attachable or independent device that connects to a bed, linen cart, or trolley via a clamp system. This bed mover is powered by batteries. Once it is attached to the bed or cart, an operator can move or steer the device. Weight capacities vary among such detachable devices (up to 2,500 lbs), as does battery life. The benefit of using these patient-transport devices is that it can be connected to many items, such as linen carts, beds, or other trolleys. The devices are not dedicated to one item. An additional advantage is that it is cheaper than a powered bed or stretcher, where the power is integrated into the bed or stretcher itself. However, the disadvantage of these devices is that they may not fit into the elevator during patient transport. To ensure maximum use, a facility should measure elevators and doorways before purchasing such devices.

To avoid the problems of detachable transport devices not fitting through doorways and onto elevators, manufacturers have designed powered, integrated systems for patient transport. This is the second type of transport available to move patients safely. The benefit of such a transport device is that you can move heavier patients with little effort. The disadvantage is that the integrated, powered transport devices are usually more expensive than the detachable devices. However, the possible reduction of injury risk makes these devices a worthwhile investment in the long term. Injuries sustained from transporting injuries can be long term and can result in disability; any technological solution that can reduce this risk is a significant one.

- Bed or stretcher with integrated system powered for transport, or nonintegrated bed mover or powered wheelchair mover
- Two or more caregivers

If powered equipment is not available, then choose the transport option that requires the fewest patient transfers. For example, a convertible chair allows transferring a patient either in a supine position or seated upright and can therefore reduce the number of potential transfers.

If using a detachable patient-transport device, make sure that the battery is fully charged and that the backup battery is also charging.

Technique 5-2

There are several considerations when transporting a patient with a detachable transport device:

1. Follow *General Directions for All Tasks.*
2. Map out the route to make sure that the bed fits through doorways and onto elevators.
3. Make sure the transport device/bed is easy to maneuver.
4. Determine how many transfers are required to accomplish the task, and minimize if possible.
5. Determine number of staff members available to assist.

6. Calculate the weight of patient plus bed to ensure elevator weight capacity and other capacities are not exceeded.
7. Determine the least physically demanding transport device when moving a patient (listed here from least to most physically demanding):
   a. Integrated powered stretcher or bed
   b. Powered wheelchair
   c. Detachable transport device with bed
   d. Convertible chair

If the bed or stretcher has integrated power, caregivers operate it using the following steps:

1. Follow *General Directions for All Tasks*.
2. Unplug the bed.
3. Release the brakes.
4. Press two buttons on the steering lever usually located at the head of the bed or stretcher.

Positioning for Bedside X-Ray

Description of Task and Associated Risks

In critical care, the patients often have diagnostic and monitoring require-ments, necessitating bedside portable X-rays. Such procedures are high-risk patient-handling tasks, due to caregiver lifting, static holding, and awkward sustained postures.

> View Video 5.2: Patient
> Positioning for Bedside X-Ray

Patient Abilities

■ Unable to assist or unable to follow instructions

Resources Required

■ Supine repositioning/lifting sling (Check the sling for metal features. Some slings have metal grommets or reinforcement stays that could interfere with radiological procedures.)
■ Lift with hanger/spreader bar that can be centered over the patient in the bed
■ One caregiver (two caregivers if the patient is uncooperative or if exces-sive lines/monitors are present)

Technique 5-3

1. Follow *General Directions for All Tasks*.
2. Place patient in supine position with head of bed at comfortable height.
3. Place supine repositioning sling beneath the patient, with the material suf-ficiently high to be above the top of the patient's head.

4. Attach the sling's upper straps via their connecting loops to the lift's hanger/spreader bar.
5. While watching the position of the patient, raise the height of the hanger bar until desired amount of separation from the bed surface is achieved.
6. Radiology technician places the photographic plate under patient's trunk.
7. Raise head of the bed to desired position.
8. After X-ray is taken, reverse steps in order to remove the photographic plate.
9. Keep sling under patient for repositioning as needed and as appropriate in caregiver's judgment.

Position for Treatment—Turning for Wound Management/Dressings

Description of Task and Associated Risks

Technique 4–6 described using a sling to turn a patient for comfort and for pressure relief. In critical care, where patients are often dependent, there are many skin treatment and access needs. Therefore, in order to turn a dependent patient to side lying with the specific intent of access to patient anatomy, an accessory with a smaller surface is recommended, because it will not block view or access. Risks to caregivers include lifting heavy weights, reaching, and sustained holds in awkward postures. Risks to patients include skin shearing.

View Video 5.3: Patient Being Turned Using the Triangle Sling

Patient Abilities

■ Unable to assist or unable to follow instructions

Resources Required

■ Ceiling-mounted or floor-based patient lift with a hanger/spreader bar
■ One–two caregivers (two needed if the patient is uncooperative)
■ Triangle or other small-surface-area sling accessory

Technique 5-4

1. Follow *General Directions for All Tasks.*
2. Patient will be in supine position with head of bed level or as close to level as tolerated by the patient.
3. Insert triangle sling by pushing down on the mattress surface to make space, and slide the sling beneath the lumbar space (low back) until the sling is through and visible on the other side of the patient. *Caution: To prevent shearing, continue to compress the mattress as sling advances and keep caregiver's hand on top of sling during placement.*
4. Attach the anchor strap securely to the bed.
5. Lower ceiling lift's spreader bar to just above patient and attach straps of sling to spreader bar.

6. Slightly bend patient's leg and cross over the knee/leg in direction patient will turn.
7. Operate the lift, raising the spreader bar, which will turn the patient. At the same time, guide patient's trunk with appropriate hand placement at shoulder/hip.
8. Patient is now on his/her side, accessible, and ready for treatment.
9. Lower patient by using ceiling-lift controls; guide patient with appropriate hand placement at shoulder/hip.
10. Detach straps from spreader bar and detach the anchor strap from the bed frame.
11. Remove sling from under patient by pushing down on the mattress surface and sliding the sling beneath the lumbar space (low back) until the sling is out on the other side of the patient.

Case Study 5-1

Ms. B is an 85-year-old woman who suffered a fall last night at home and was admitted to the hospital. She is cognitively impaired, has bruising on her face, and has a possible broken right arm and right hip. Her vital signs are currently stable; however, Ms. B. needs oxygen per nasal cannula to maintain adequate oxygen saturation levels. She also has intravenous fluids running into her left forearm.

5.3

Positioning for wound management/ dressings

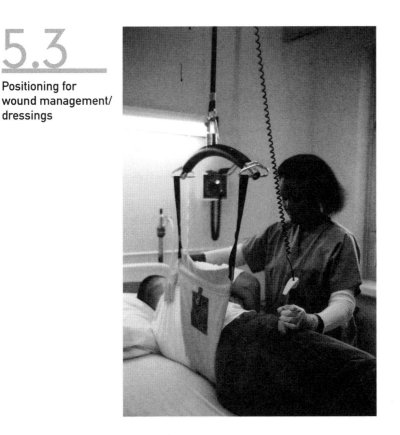

Ms. B was admitted to the critical care unit because of her age and potential injuries. X-rays of her arm and hip have been ordered for this morning. The X-ray department is located at the other end of the hospital and is four floors down. Ms. B.'s caregiver does not have much help on this case because most of the health care team members are responding to a code at the moment. The equipment options available to the caregiver are these:

1. A mobile chair that converts from supine to seated
2. A lateral transfer aid
3. A stretcher
4. A floor-based lift
5. A powered bed

Discussion Questions:

1. Given the medical condition of Ms. B, which technological choice would be most appropriate in this case and why?
2. What are the determining factors that led you to your decision?
3. What preparation/assessment needs to be done prior to moving Ms. B?

Case Study 5-2

Mrs. G is a 63-year-old woman who arrived in the emergency room with chief complaints of shortness of breath and chest pain. She is being admitted to the Cardiac Intensive Care Unit with the diagnosis of "rule out myocardial infarction." Her initial chest X-ray reveals evidence of heart failure (HF). Upon admission to the unit, Mrs. G.'s physical exam reveals an obese female, approximately 5 feet tall, weighing 200 lbs. Her heart rate is 100–106 and regular in rhythm. She has bilateral lower-limb edema. Her pulse oximetry is 93% with bilateral crackles noted on inspiration. Mrs. G is mildly sedated because she is receiving mechanical ventilation support, but she is cooperative and responsive when awake. It appears Mrs. G is fatigued, and it is difficult for her to move in bed because of the endotracheal tube/ventilator and two intravenous lines in her right arm.

Among the many orders regarding Mrs. G's care, she is to receive a diuretic medication for excess fluid removal to treat her HF, Foley catheter insertion, and bedside, portable, follow-up chest X-ray. You need to (1) place her Foley catheter, and (2) work with radiology to obtain the portable chest X-ray. You have a ceiling-mounted lift and the related sling accessories in the ICU room assigned to Mrs. G.

Discussion Questions:

1. What is the *most important* assessment factor in determining Mrs. G's need for assistance in patient handling? Explain your answer.
2. Practice explaining the two procedures to the patient. Pretending you are Mrs. G, critique the clarity and length of each other's explanations.

3. What types of equipment are appropriate for completing these handling tasks?
4. If a coworker suggests Mrs. G. doesn't need any equipment assistance and the co-worker wants to assist you in performing the tasks, solely on a manual basis, what is the best action for you to take?

Post-Test Questions

5-1. You are the nurse caring for a female patient who is on a ventilator and in a coma. You will be inserting a Foley catheter. What is the best choice of equipment for this task?
   a. Use a sling that will lift and support limb(s) for procedure.
   b. Have two health care workers hold both legs in position for procedure.
   c. Have one other health care worker hold both legs in position for procedure.
   d. None of the above are correct.

5-2. What patient-care task has the potential for staff injury in critical care?
   a. Repositioning, "boosting up" in bed
   b. Turning patient
   c. Positioning patient for procedures or exams
   d. All of the above

5-3. Sustained holding of a patient's leg has been identified as a high-risk task in critical care. Why is it a physically demanding task?
   a. Because of the weight of the leg
   b. Because of the size of the leg
   c. Because of the awkward posture that the caregiver adopts when holding the leg
   d. Because of all of the above

5-4. Which of the following statements is *not* true?
   a. There are two types of patient-transport devices: detachable and integrated.
   b. Integrated patient-transport devices are those that can attach to a bed, trolley, or cart.
   c. Integrated devices are typically more expensive than detachable devices.
   d. Patient transport devices are a good option because they can reduce the push forces involved in moving beds, carts, or trolleys.

5-5. You are the nurse caring for a patient in the intensive care unit. This patient will be transported to another floor in his bed. He has chest tubes and a ventilator. What is the best method for transferring this patient?
   a. Bed mover to move bed
   b. One health care worker for ventilator
   c. One health care worker for chest tubes
   d. All of the above

References

Waters, T. R., Nelson, A. L., & Proctor, C. (2007). Patient handling tasks with high risk for musculoskeletal disorders in critical care. *Critical Care Nursing Clinics of North America, 19,* 131–143.

Waters, T. R. (2007). When is it safe to manually lift a patient? The revised NIOSH lifting equation provides support for recommended weight limits. *American Journal of Nursing, 107*(8), 53–58.

Additional Reading

Baptiste, A., McCleerey, M., Matz, M., & Evitt, C. (2008). Proper sling selection and application while using patient lifts. *Rehabilitation Nursing, 33*(1), 24–34.

Baptiste, A. (2008). Safe client movement and handling. In D. Fell-Carlson (Ed.), *Working safely in health care: A practical guide* (pp. 94–145). Clifton Park, NY: Delmar Learning.

Baptiste, A. (2007). Technology solutions for high risk tasks in critical care. *Critical Care Nursing Clinics of North America 19,* 177–186.

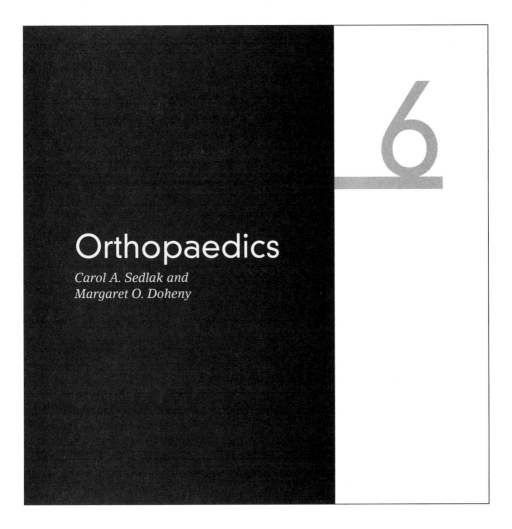

Orthopaedics

Carol A. Sedlak and
Margaret O. Doheny

Description of Setting

The term *orthopaedics* is drawn from the Greek words *orthos* (straight) and *paidos* (child). Agnes Hunt is known as the Florence Nightingale of orthopaedic nursing. She had a childhood deformity that motivated her to open a training school for orthopaedic nurses (Schoen, 2000). The speciality of orthopaedic nursing focuses on prevention and care of musculoskeletal disorders (Salmond, 2002). The current professional nursing association for orthopaedic nurses is the National Association of Orthopaedic Nurses (NAON), which was formally established in 1980. The mission of the National Association of Orthopaedic Nurses is to advance the specialty of orthopaedic nursing through excellence in research, education, and nursing practice (NAON, n.d.). In 2006 the NAON Safe Patient Handling and Movement Task Force was developed. NAON's work on this important initiative was intended to provide evidence-based, practical ergonomic methods for safe patient handling of orthopaedic patients to prevent injuries for nurses, patients, and health care workers (Sedlak, 2006).

Unique Challenges to Providing Safe Patient Handling in this Setting

This chapter describes high-risk tasks that are performed by nurses working with patients who have orthopaedic limitations. The goal is to prevent musculoskeletal injuries associated with patient-handling tasks. Orthopaedic patients may have limited ability to flex, extend, and position themselves and may have hardware, casts, vests, braces, and other apparatuses attached that limit mobility and add to patient weight. For this reason, NAON developed orthopaedic algorithms to ensure safety for both caregiver and patient (NAON, in press).

High-Risk Tasks

The five high-risk tasks in this chapter include the following:

1. Turning a patient in bed side to side (patient with orthopaedic impairments)
2. Vertical transfer of a postoperative total hip replacement (THR) patient
3. Vertical transfer of a patient with a cast/splint on upper extremity: immobilized arm
4. Vertical transfer of a patient with a cast/splint on lower extremity: immobilized leg
5. Ambulation

A specifically developed table for lifting and holding legs and/or arms will be discussed.

Objectives

Describe the unique challenges associated with safe patient handling in orthopaedic patient populations.

1. Identify high-risk patient-handling tasks on orthopaedic units.
2. Delineate the number of caregivers, types of equipment, and techniques for performing each high-risk patient-handling task safely.

Pre-Test Questions

6-1. The high-risk tasks that have been identified by orthopaedic nurses are these:
    a. Turning the patient with orthopaedic impairments in bed side to side
    b. Vertically transferring a postoperative total hip replacement patient
    c. Vertically transferring a patient with a cast/splint on upper extremity
    d. All of the above

6-2. When preparing to move an orthopaedic patient, what is the first step?
   a. Obtain lifting equipment.
   b. Assess the patient.
   c. Select the correct algorithm.
   d. Enlist help of peers.

6-3. When planning to complete a vertical transfer of a cooperative patient with an immobilized arm who is able to partially bear weight on the lower extremities, what is the best way to transfer the patient?
   a. Using a floor-based or ceiling-mounted patient lift with a sling
   b. Using caregiver standby assistance
   c. Using manual stand-and-pivot technique
   d. Using a power-assisted lift with two caregivers

6-4. When planning to complete a vertical transfer of an uncooperative patient with an immobilized leg, the best choice of action for the transfer is to:
   a. Use mobility aids as prescribed by the team.
   b. Use a floor-based or ceiling-mounted patient lift with at least three caregivers.
   c. Assess the total weight of the extremity.
   d. Not ambulate the patient.

6-5. Using the lifting/holding chart for determining when an assistive device is needed for lifting an arm or a leg, the maximum weight of the extremity allowed for a two-handed hold less than one minute is:
   a. 4.6 lbs
   b. 7.1 lbs
   c. 9.7 lbs
   d. 22.2 lbs

6-6. When moving a patient with an upper-extremity cast or splint, which of the following should you assess prior to the transfer of a patient?
   a. Level of pain, fatigue, ability to cooperate
   b. Attitude, mental status, weight
   c. Age, height, level of pain
   d. Ability to cooperate, weight, age

General Directions for All Tasks

1. Complete *Assessment Criteria and Care Plan* for patient. Key assessment factors include physical ability to assist, ability to follow instructions, and cooperation. *Note: Weight and height may trigger use of bariatric algorithms.*
2. Review the algorithm for the high-risk patient-handling task to be performed and determine the number of caregivers, types of equipment, and techniques for performing each high-risk patient-handling task safely. If no algorithm exists, use the techniques described in this book to guide practice.
3. Check the weight capacity of the equipment to be sure it is able to handle the patient's weight.

4. Remove obstacles to performing the patient-handling tasks. Obstacles include too little room to maneuver the equipment, equipment stored on the floor posing a stumbling hazard, or inability to perform the activity without threats to patient dignity (e.g., lack of privacy). You may need to remove chairs or bed tables, separate beds, move floor-based equipment, and ask visitors to leave.

5. Make sure selected equipment is in good working order. If the equipment is battery operated, check that the battery is charged. Verify that the appropriate slings and attachments are available. Review safe operation of the equipment, including location of emergency buttons or manual controls for the event of a power failure.

6. Ensure sufficient caregivers are available to help, as specified in the algorithm.

7. Make sure beds are adjusted to caregiver's waist/elbow height before performing bed-related patient-handling tasks.

8. Explain the procedure to the patient and assisting caregivers.

9. Wear gloves according to proper infection-control practices and facility policies.

Turning an Orthopaedic Patient in Bed (Side to Side)

Description of Task and Associated Risks

This algorithm provides various techniques for turning a patient side to side in bed when orthopaedic impairments are present (e.g., patient has halo vest or external fixators). This is the first step when beginning to move an orthopaedic patient. Risks to the caregiver include reaching, pushing/pulling, and lifting heavy weights. Risks to the patient include skin shearing. Refer to Appendix A, Algorithm 15.

View Video 6.1: Turning a Patient Wearing a Halo Vest in Bed Using a Ceiling Lift

Patient Abilities

■ Unable to perform task independently

Resources Required

■ Floor-based or ceiling-mounted patient lift or bed-assisted technology, such as turning clips (devices that attach directly to the bed sheet to facilitate turning a patient in bed), patient repositioning systems, ceiling-mounted patient lifts. or air bladders (built into bed surfaces and specialized mattresses; as one side deflates, the other side inflates, thus turning the patient on his/her side)

■ Side rail or repositioning pole

■ Two caregivers

Technique 6-1

1. Follow *General Directions for All Tasks.*
2. Maintain orthopaedic precautions as prescribed by physician such as THR.
3. If the patient is not cooperative, a floor-based or ceiling-mounted patient lift or bed-assistive technology is needed.
4. If the patient is cooperative but cannot assist, then use a mechanical device or bed-assistive technology.
5. Use a sling with the floor-based or ceiling-mounted patient lift (See Helpful Hints: Slings.)

Helpful Hints: Slings

Selection of the appropriate sling accessory for movement/lift/transfer must include the following considerations:

- Deciding to transfer patient in sitting vs. supine position—choosing correct functionality of the sling
- Selecting appropriate size
- Maintaining alignment of the affected body part(s) according to preoperative/postoperative guidelines.
  - Consider the patient's body size, shape and features (e.g., very large abdominal girth limiting degree of hip flexion)
  - Features of sling:
    - Where material covers the patient
    - Strap options for seated slings—the length of material for strap supports of the lower extremities can often be modified by selecting differing loop attachment points of the sling onto the hanger bar (providing more material length will allow lower extremity to be in less flexed position)
    - Seated slings' back height can vary from supporting whole trunk and head to covering pelvis/waist only. When upper extremities are involved, consider height of the sling—high-back slings will wrap around and enclose an upper extremity, whereas a low-back sling will allow upper extremity to be free.

6. For any patient who is at risk for pressure ulcers, use care to prevent shearing force when using any device. Friction-reducing devices (FRDs) will reduce shearing forces.
7. If alignment/positioning guidelines cannot be met with available sling accessory, transfer patient supine with sheet-style sling or antifriction methods, then sit patient upright.

Vertical Transfer of a Postoperative Total Hip Replacement (THR) Patient

Description of Task and Associated Risks

This algorithm provides various methods for moving a patient with a THR from a supine position to sitting on the side of the bed. The patient must be able to sit on the edge of the bed and maintain THR precautions. If the caregiver is required to lift more than 35 lbs of a patient's weight, mechanical assistance is needed. The patient's pain, level of fatigue, and ability to cooperate must be considered by the caregiver before moving the patient. Refer to Appendix A, Algorithm 16.

View Video 6.2: Vertical Transfer of a THR Patient Using a Sit-to-Stand Lift

Patient Abilities

■ Variable ability to cooperate, bear weight, assist, maintain THR precautions, tolerate seated position, and shift weight in seated position

Resources Required

■ Floor-based or ceiling-mounted patient lift
■ Slings
■ Mobility aids such as walker, cane, crutches
■ One–two caregivers, depending on the patient's ability to move

Technique 6-2

1. Follow *General Directions for All Tasks*.
2. Maintain THR precautions as prescribed.
3. Assess if the patient is cooperative. If not, use a floor-based or ceiling-mounted patient lift with two caregivers.
4. Select and inspect the appropriate sling size and type for the patient. Follow the manufacturer's directions for applying sling. Technique to apply sling is usually rolling the patient from side to side (see Appendix A, Algorithm 15). Position patient on back after sling is inserted under patient.
5. The nursing decision about whether to remove the sling or leave it under the patient should be made considering the patient's skin integrity, tolerance of the sling surface, and length of time in the chair. If the patient is remaining in the chair for an extended period of time or has been transferred to the bed, remove the transfer sling.
6. If the patient is cooperative and can fully bear weight, a mobility aid such as a walker, cane, or crutches is needed. Stand by for safety as needed.
7. If the patient is cooperative and can partially bear weight, a stand-and-pivot technique is needed with a gait/transfer belt. Alternatively, use a powered standing assist with one caregiver.
8. Check manufacturer's recommendations regarding brake application for all equipment.

Vertical Transfer of a Patient with Cast or Splint on Upper Extremity

Description of Task and Associated Risks

This algorithm provides various methods for moving a patient with a cast or splint on the upper extremity. The caregiver needs to assess the patient's level of pain, fatigue, and ability to cooperate and support the limb while the patient moves. Risks to the caregiver include lifting heavy weights, making awkward postures, and twisting. Refer to Appendix A, Algorithm 17.

> View Video 6.3: Transfer of a Patient With an Arm Splint/Cast Using a Friction Reducing Device and Pivot Disk

Patient Abilities

- Variable ability to cooperate, assist, and bear weight

Resources Required

- Floor-based or ceiling-mounted patient lift
- Pivot disc
- FRD
- Sling
- Mobility aid such as walker, cane, or crutches
- One–two caregivers, depending on the patient's ability to move.

Technique 6-3

1. Follow *General Directions for All Tasks*.
2. If the patient is not cooperative, use a floor-based or ceiling-mounted patient lift with two caregivers.
3. Select and inspect the appropriate sling size and type for the patient. Follow the manufacturer's directions for applying the sling. The technique to apply a sling is usually rolling the patient from side to side (see Appendix A, Algorithm 15). Position patient on his/her back after sling is inserted.
4. If the patient is cooperative and can partially bear weight, position the patient at the side of the bed.
   a. To move to the side of the bed, the patient must move from supine to a sitting position. The patient will need to shift his or her seated weight and move by lifting one buttock and moving toward the edge of the bed, repeating in an alternate fashion until sitting on the edge of the bed. Use of an FRD is helpful for this maneuver.
   b. If the patient requires the help of a caregiver and the amount of assistance from the caregiver exceeds lifting 35 lbs of the patient's weight, use a floor-based or ceiling-mounted patient lift to achieve a sitting position at the edge of the bed.

5. Help the patient to a standing position by using the manual stand-and-pivot technique (with or without a gait/transfer belt) or by using a stand-and-pivot device or a powered standing-assistive device.
   ■ When a patient has an impaired upper extremity, the caregiver may need to support the limb while the patient attempts to move to a sitting position. Refer to Appendix A, Clinical Tool #1 (Lifting and Holding Legs or Arms in an Orthopaedic Setting). When a caregiver must lift a leg or arm, be sure that the weight of the limb being lifted does not exceed the strength capability of the caregiver. Use this table to determine whether a specific lift or hold of a limb is acceptable and whether some type of lift- or hold-assist device is needed.
6. If the patient can bear weight fully, caregiver assistance is not needed. Stand by for safety as needed.

Vertical Transfer of a Patient with Cast or Splint on Lower Extremity

Description of Task and Associated Risks

View Video 6.4: Transfer of a Patient With a Long Leg Splint Using a Floor-Based Lift

This algorithm provides various methods for moving a patient with a cast or splint on the lower extremity, which requires the caregiver to support the limb while the patient moves. Risks to caregivers include lifting heavy loads, awkward postures, and pushing/pulling. The risk to the patient is falling. Refer to Appendix A, Algorithm 17.

Patient Abilities

■ Variable ability to cooperate, assist, and bear weight

Resources Required

■ Floor-based or ceiling-mounted patient lift
■ Slings
■ Mobility aids such as walker, cane, crutches
■ One–two caregivers, depending on the patient's ability to move

Technique 6-4

1. Follow *General Directions for All Tasks*
2. If the patient is not cooperative, use a floor-based or ceiling-mounted patient lift with two caregivers.
3. Select and inspect the appropriate sling size and type for the patient. Follow manufacturer's directions for applying sling. The technique to apply a sling is usually rolling the patient from side to side (see Appendix A, Algorithm 15). Patient should be positioned on back after sling is inserted.

4. If the patient is cooperative and can partially bear weight with the lower extremities, the patient must be positioned at the side of the bed.

   a. To move to the side of the bed, the patient must move from a supine to a sitting position. The patient will need to shift his or her seated weight and move by lifting one buttock and moving toward the edge of the bed, repeating in an alternate fashion until sitting on the edge of the bed. Use of an FRD is helpful for this maneuver.

   b. If the patient requires the help of a caregiver and the amount of assistance from the caregiver exceeds lifting over 35 lbs/16kg of the patient's weight, then use a floor-based or ceiling-mounted lift to achieve a sitting position at the edge of the bed.

5. The patient is assisted by one or two caregivers to a standing position by using the manual stand-and-pivot technique (with or without a gait/transfer belt) or by using a stand-and-pivot device or a powered sit-to-stand lift.

   With an impaired lower extremity, the caregiver may need to support the limb while the patient attempts to move to a sitting position. Use Appendix A, Clinical Tool #1 to determine whether a specific lift or hold of a limb is acceptable and whether some type of lift- or hold-assist device is needed.

6. If the patient can bear weight fully, caregiver assistance is not needed. Stand by for safety as needed.

Ambulation

Description of Task and Associated Risks

In health care, weight-bearing status is often used to describe the amount of lower-extremity weight bearing that the patient can or has performed. It is generally a reflection of muscular strength of the lower extremities. In the case of the orthopaedic patient, weight-bearing status is prescribed by the health care provider and is based on the load the musculoskeletal system will safely tolerate following orthopaedic surgery or injury. This algorithm provides various methods to ambulate an orthopaedic patient, an intervention critical to reducing postoperative complications. If the patient is unable to bear weight on the lower extremities, this activity is contraindicated. Refer to Appendix A, Algorithm 18.

> View Video 6.5: Ambulation of a Patient Using a Ceiling Lift

Patient Abilities

- Variable ability to cooperate, assist, bear weight, and grasp with one hand, with variable upper-extremity strength

Safety risks are an important concern before ambulating a patient. If the patient is determined to be at risk for falls, then the caregiver is also at risk when assisting a patient to prevent falling. The caregiver should take fall precautions and use an assistive device, such as a walking sling. The caregiver should assess the benefits and risks to walking to determine the course of action to be taken to promote ambulation.

Resources Required

- Ceiling-mounted or floor-based patient lift with ambulation sling
- Mobility aids such as walker, cane, crutches
- One–two caregivers depending on the patient's ability to move
  - During any patient-handling task, if the caregiver is required to lift more than 35 lbs/16kg of a patient's weight, then the patient should be considered fully dependent and an assistive device should be used.

Technique 6-5

1. Follow *General Directions for All Tasks.*
2. Maintain the affected extremity in immobilization/alignment.
3. If the patient cannot bear weight with the lower extremity, do not ambulate.
4. If the patient is cooperative and can fully or partially bear weight with the lower extremities and is a low safety risk, then the caregiver stands by for safety as needed and uses mobility aids prescribed (crutches, walker, cane).
5. If the patient is a high safety risk and is unable to grasp and use the upper extremity, then a ceiling-mounted or floor-based patient lift is needed with one or two caregivers.
6. If the patient is high risk for safety but does have upper-extremity strength, then a ceiling-mounted or floor-based patient lift with an ambulation sling is needed.

Lifting and Holding Legs or Arms in an Orthopaedic Setting

Description of Task and Associated Risks

In addition to the four orthopaedic algorithms described, often when orthopaedic care is being provided, the caregiver must lift or hold a limb in place while some type of treatment is being provided, such as cast application. When a caregiver must lift a leg or arm, it is important to make sure that the weight of the limb being lifted does not exceed the strength capability of the caregiver. An ergonomic tool (see Appendix A, Clinical Tool #1) has been developed to assist caregivers in determining whether a specific lift or hold of a limb is acceptable and whether some type of lift- or hold-assist device is needed. Risks to caregivers include lifting heavy weights and awkward postures. For lifts of limbs with casts, an alternate method has been presented for assessing whether a manual lift is acceptable or not.

Appendix A, Clinical Tool #1 shows the calculation of the average weight for an adult patient's leg and arm as a function of whole-body mass, ranging from slim to morbidly obese body type. Weights are presented both in pounds (lbs) and metric (kg) units. Maximum lift-and-hold loads were calculated based on 75th-percentile shoulder flexion strength and endurance capability for U.S. adult females, where the maximum weight for a one-handed lift is 11.1 lbs and a two-handed lift, 22.2lbs. Appendix A, Clinical Tool #2 shows safe holding and lifting limits of limbs for persons with casts.

Case Study 6-1

Mrs. Price is 68 years old and is a 1-day post-op right total hip replacement (THR) patient. The physician wrote an order for her to be out of bed and begin ambulation. Through the postoperative night, she has requested pain medication and states her pain is now 3/10. She is cooperative and is eager to progress in her care. She has been able to assist with turning from side to side using a positioning device. She has maintained THR precautions. You have reviewed Mrs. Price's ambulation orders and note that she can partially bear weight on her right leg.

Discussion Questions

1. What personnel and equipment will you need to assist Mrs. Price with a vertical transfer?
2. What are the THR precautions you need to follow?
3. What are the weight parameters to follow when supporting the affected limb?
4. When would you consider using FRDs?
5. How would you use a powered sit-to-stand lift?

Post-Test Questions

6-1. The high-risk tasks that have been identified by orthopaedic nurses are these:
   a. Turning the patient with orthopaedic impairments in bed side to side
   b. Vertically transferring of a postoperative total hip replacement patient
   c. Vertically transferring a patient with a cast/splint on upper extremity
   d. All of the above
6-2. When preparing to move an orthopaedic patient, what is the first step?
   a. Obtain lifting equipment.
   b. Assess the patient.
   c. Select the correct algorithm.
   d. Enlist help of peers.
6-3. When planning to complete a vertical transfer of a cooperative patient with an immobilized arm who is able to partially bear weight on the lower extremities, what is the best way to transfer the patient?
   a. Using a floor-based or ceiling-mounted patient lift with a sling
   b. Using caregiver standby assistance
   c. Using manual stand-and-pivot technique
   d. Using a power-assisted lift with two caregivers

6-4. When planning to complete a vertical transfer of an uncooperative patient with an immobilized leg, the best choice of action for the transfer is to:
   a. Use mobility aids as prescribed by the team.
   b. Use a floor-based or ceiling-mounted patient lift with at least three caregivers.
   c. Assess the total weight of the extremity.
   d. Not ambulate the patient.

6-5. Using the lifting/holding chart for determining when an assistive device is needed for lifting an arm or a leg, the maximum weight of the extremity allowed for a two-handed hold less than one minute is:
   a. 4.6 lbs
   b. 7.1 lbs
   c. 9.7 lbs
   d. 22.2 lbs

6-6. When moving a patient with an upper-extremity cast or splint, which of the following should you assess prior to the transfer?
   a. Patient's level of pain, fatigue, ability to cooperate
   b. Patient's attitude, mental status, weight
   c. Patient's age, height, level of pain
   d. Patient's ability to cooperate, weight, age

References

National Association of Orthopaedic Nurses (NAON). (n.d.). Mission and philosophy. Retrieved 18 November 2008, from http://www.orthonurse.org/AboutNAON/MissionandPhilosophy/tabid/291/Default.aspx

National Association of Orthopaedic Nurses (NAON). (In press). Safe patient handling. *Orthopaedic Nursing, 28*(2), supplement.

Salmond, S. W. (2002). Orthopaedic wellness. In A. B. Maher, S.W. Salmond, and T.A. Pellino (Eds.), *Orthopaedic Nursing* (3rd ed.) (pp. 1–26). Philadelphia, PA: W.B. Saunders.

Schoen, D. C. (2000). *Adult Orthopaedic Nursing.* Philadelphia, PA: Lippincott.

Sedlak, C.A. (2006). Guest editorial. Nursing safety: NAON's role in preventing workplace musculoskeletal injury. *Orthopaedic Nursing, 25*(6), 354–355.

Additional Reading

Chaffin, D. B., Anderson, G. B. J., & Martin, B. J. (1999). *Occupational biomechanics* (3rd ed.). New York: Wiley & Sons.

Nelson, A. L. (Ed.) (2006). *Safe patient handling and movement: A practical guide for health care professionals.* New York: Springer.

Nelson, A., Baptiste, A. (September 30, 2004). Evidence-based practices for safe patient handling and movement. *Online Journal of Issues in Nursing.* Vol. 9 No. 3, Manuscript 3. Retrieved December 10, 2008, from http://www.nursingworld.org/MainMenuCategories/ANAMarketplace/ANAPeriodicals/OJIN/TableofContents/Volume92004/No3Sept04/EvidenceBasedPractices.aspx

Pheasant, S. (1992). *Bodyspace.* London: Taylor & Francis.

Rohmert, W. (1973a). Problems of determination of rest allowances. Part 1: Use of modern methods to evaluate stress and strain in static muscular work. *Applied Ergonomics, 4*(2), 91–95.

Rohmert, W. (1973b). Problems of determination of rest allowances. Part 2: Determining rest allowances in different human tasks. *Applied Ergonomics, 4*(3), 158–162.

Waters, T. (2007). When is it safe to manually lift a patient? *American Journal of Nursing, 107*(8), 53–59.

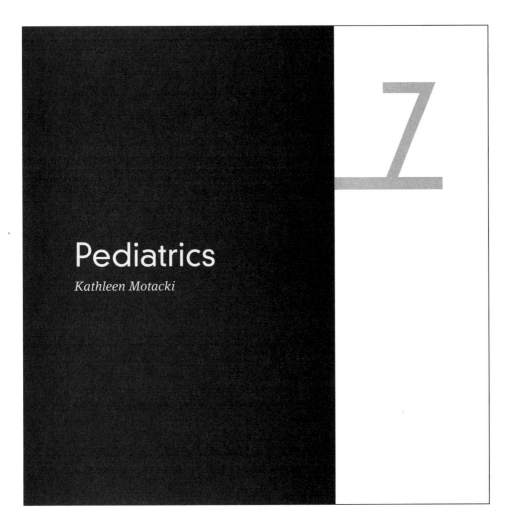

Pediatrics

Kathleen Motacki

Description of Setting

Pediatrics is a specialty area involving children. There are many practice settings for the pediatric population, including acute care, rehabilitation, perioperative, dialysis, outpatient, schools, home care, and primary care.

Unique Challenges to Providing Safe Patient Handling in this Setting

There is a misconception that patient handling in pediatrics is not risky because the patients are small. Evidence supports the safety of manual patient handling for weights up to 35 lbs or 15.9 kg (Waters, 2007). Pediatric patients can and do exceed this weight limit, especially adolescents, who can weigh as much as adults. Furthermore, unique factors in pediatrics make other patient-handling tasks high risk, based on their sustained awkward postures, excessive bending, twisting, reaching, and long duration. Patient-handling equipment comes in all sizes (Department of Veterans Affairs (VHA) VISN 8 Patient Safety Center of Inquiry, 2001). Although caregivers may be familiar with adult-sized equipment, they must be aware that devices and supporting slings need to be appropriate for children. Furthermore, when caring for the pediatric patient, the caregiver must keep in mind that children are unpredictable at times and may not always be cooperative, which significantly increases caregiver risk.

High-Risk Tasks

The high-risk tasks that have been identified for infant, child, and adolescent patients are listed below:

1. Feeding baby or child
2. Putting on a body jacket
3. Lifting a toddler from a playpen

Objectives

1. Describe the unique challenges associated with safe patient handling in pediatric patient populations.
2. Identify high-risk patient-handling tasks in pediatric units.
3. Delineate the number of caregivers, types of equipment, and techniques for performing each high-risk patient-handling task safely.

Pre-Test Questions

7-1. How many kilograms should a pediatric patient weigh to trigger the use of lifting equipment?
  a. 16
  b. 20
  c. 25
  d. 26
7-2. How many caregivers are needed to lift an uncooperative pediatric patient who weighs 50 kg?
  a. One
  b. Two
  c. Three
  d. Four
7-3. When you are lifting a comatose male teenager (adult size, adult weight, and adult height) from bed to wheelchair, what should you do?
  a. Use appropriate adult algorithm for this transfer.
  b. Use pediatric algorithm.
  c. Allow patient to remain in bed.
  d. None of the above.

7-4. If a child weighs more than 30 kg and needs to be lifted from the floor, which of the following is most appropriate?
  a. Use a floor-based patient lift.
  b. Lift the child alone.
  c. Lift the child with two caregivers.
  d. None of the above.

7-5. You are caring for a 12-year-old boy who needs to be transferred to his wheelchair from his bed. You are unable to locate the appropriate size of sling for the child. What is the first thing that you should do?
  a. Use whatever sling is available on the unit.
  b. Manually lift him into his wheelchair.
  c. Obtain a sling that is the proper size for the child.
  d. None of the above.

7-6. You are a new caregiver working in the adolescent unit. During the hospital orientation, you are educated on the adult safe-lifting equipment available. One of your patients requires a lift to get him out of bed. The equipment on the pediatric floor is different from the one you have been trained on. What do you do?
  a. Inform your charge caregiver that you have not been trained on this piece of equipment.
  b. Do the lift with the unfamiliar equipment.
  c. Ask a coworker to complete the lift until you receive training.
  d. Both *a* and *c* are correct.

7-7. The best way to evaluate the size of a sling for a patient in pediatrics is to:
  a. Use an adult small size
  b. Measure the child as per manufacturer's protocol
  c. Assume it is safe to manually lift children
  d. All of the above

General Directions for All Tasks

1. Complete *Assessment Criteria and Care Plan* for patient. Key assessment factors include physical ability to assist, ability to follow instructions, and cooperation. *Note: Weight and height may trigger use of bariatric algorithms.*
2. Review the algorithm for the high-risk patient-handling task to be performed and determine the number of caregivers, types of equipment, and techniques for performing each high-risk patient-handling task safely. If no algorithm exists, use the techniques described in this book to guide practice.
3. Check the weight capacity of the equipment to be sure it is able to handle the patient's weight.
4. Remove obstacles to performing the patient-handling tasks. Obstacles include too little room to maneuver the equipment, equipment stored on the floor posing a stumbling hazard, or inability to perform the activity without threats to patient dignity (e.g., lack of privacy). You may need to remove chairs or bed tables, separate beds, move floor-based equipment, and ask visitors to leave.

5. Make sure selected equipment is in good working order. If the equipment is battery operated, check that the battery is charged. Verify that the appropriate slings and attachments are available. Review safe operation of the equipment, including location of emergency buttons or manual controls for the event of a power failure.
6. Ensure sufficient caregivers are available to help, as specified in the algorithm.
7. Make sure beds are adjusted to caregiver's waist/elbow height before performing bed-related patient-handling tasks.
8. Explain the procedure to the patient and assisting caregivers.
9. Wear gloves according to proper infection-control practices and facility policies.

Feeding a Baby

Description of Task and Associated Risks

When babies are in hospitals, their illnesses often contribute to longer feeding times. An example is if the baby has had cleft lip or cleft palate repair, or if the infant is premature and has sucking and swallowing problems. The feeding task is typically of long duration and may involve static postures, which contribute to caregiver risk.

View Video 7.1: Feeding a Baby

Patient Abilities

■ Unable to assist

Resources Required

■ One adult-sized chair
■ One caregiver
■ Feeding supplies

Technique 7-1

1. Follow *General Directions for All Tasks*.
2. Make sure bottle and burping pad are near.
3. Feed baby on one arm for 5–10 minutes; burp baby.
4. Switch baby to other arm for 5–10 minutes.
5. Continue with this method until feeding time has ended.

7.1

Holding baby on right arm during feeding

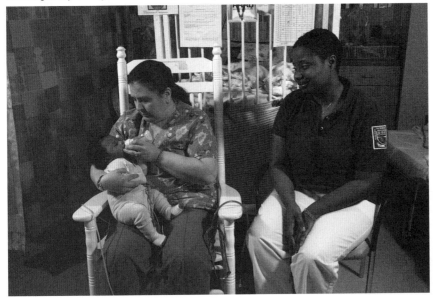

7.2

Holding baby in burping position

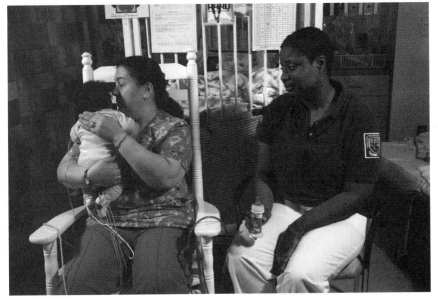

7.3

Holding baby on left arm during feeding

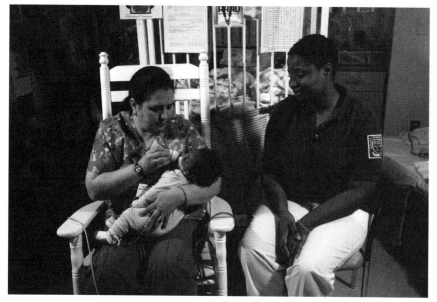

Feeding Children

Description of Task and Associated Risks

Another task that is performed in pediatrics is feeding children. Often when children are ill, they need assistance with feeding. For example, the child who has sustained a brain injury may need to relearn the task of chewing and swallowing. It is essential that during feeding the child is in an upright position.

Feeding can be high risk to the caregiver because it is characterized as a task of long duration, performed in awkward positions, with excessive reaching. To minimize this risk, the caregiver should avoid using child-sized chairs when performing feeding tasks. The child should be placed in a wheelchair or high chair, and the caregiver's chair should be even with the patient so there is no reaching. Depending on the situation, either an adult-sized chair or a height-adjustable chair can be used to minimize risk. When feeding a toddler, for example, if the toddler is in bed, the caregiver should be sitting even with bed level. Avoid reaching to perform the task.

Patient Abilities

■ Unable to assist

Resources Required

- One adult-sized chair or height-adjustable stool
- One caregiver
- Feeding supplies

Technique 7-2

1. Follow *General Directions for All Tasks*.
2. Position child's body at same height as caregiver's body.
3. Regardless of whether the child is fed in a highchair, wheelchair, chair, or bed, avoid excessive reach and change positions frequently.

Caregiver feeding child on face-to-face level, caregiver on adult-sized chair

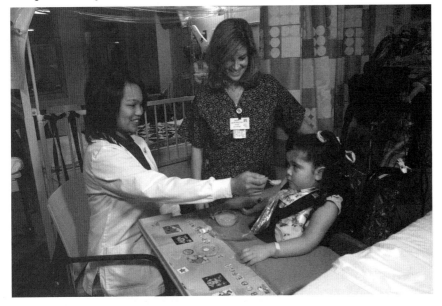

Placing a Body Jacket

Description of Task and Associated Risks

A body jacket is used for the child who has sustained a spinal cord injury (SCI) or one who has a disability such as severe scoliosis. The purpose of a body jacket is to maintain proper body alignment while the patient is out of bed.

Patient-handling tasks for the pediatric patient in a body jacket are challenging. The body jacket is made out of very hard material that adds additional weight to each task performed. Further, the rigidity of the jacket limits patient mobility, increasing dependence on the caregiver (which increases exposure to other high-risk tasks associated with patient transfers, bathing, etc.). Providing patient handling for a child in a body jacket is considered high risk due to the weight lifted, sustained awkward positions used to work around the jacket, and excessive reaching.

Patient Abilities

- Unable to assist

Resources Required

- Child's body jacket
- Two caregivers (three needed if patient is not cooperative)

Technique 7-3

1. Follow *General Directions for All Tasks*.
2. Position one caregiver on each side of patient.
3. First caregiver rolls child to one side.
4. First caregiver applies body jacket under child.
5. Both caregivers should turn child to back, then to opposite side.
6. Second caregiver applies body jacket to other side.
7. Fasten tabs on front of body jacket.

One caregiver on each side of child's bed, one caregiver placing body jacket on bed

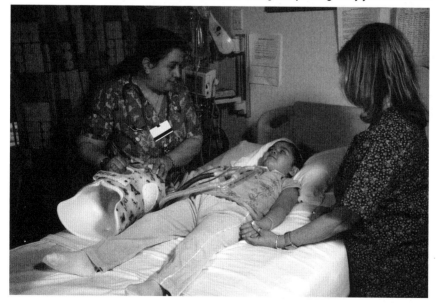

7.6

First caregiver turning patient toward second caregiver

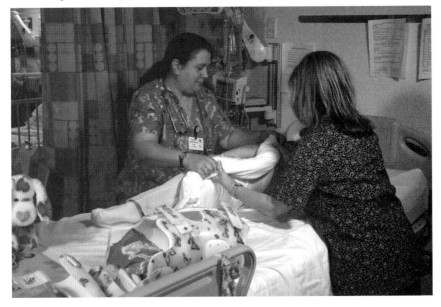

7.7

Second caregiver placing body jacket on child

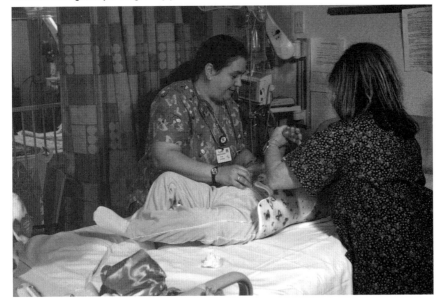

Lifting a Toddler Out of a Playpen

Description of Task and Associated Risks

Playpens are used in pediatric rehabilitation units. This task is performed with the toddler at or near floor level. That is one of the reasons why it is considered high risk. As discussed in chapter 2, when a patient who is unable to assist is on the floor, the caregiver should always use a lifting device. The same holds true when in the pediatric setting.

View Video 7.2: Lifting a Toddler out of a Playpen

The musculoskeletal risk associated with manually lifting a toddler out of a playpen increases based on the frequency this task is performed in a given workday. The task involves a heavy weight lifted with outstretched arms. Holding a weight in this position is much harder than holding a weight close to the body, and the 35-lb weight limit under ideal conditions (Waters, 2007) actually is an overestimate of safe weight limit for manual lifting because the task is performed under less-than-ideal conditions (outstretched arms). At times it is hard for caregivers to use patient-handling equipment for small children because they feel manual lifting meets the patient's need for human contact and affection. However, using the patient-handling equipment is safer and does not rule out holding the patient post-lift to meet the patient's needs.

Patient Abilities

- Unable to walk or stand
- Unable to cooperate

Resources Required

- Floor-based patient lift
- One caregiver

Technique 7-4

1. Follow *General Directions for All Tasks*.
2. Select the appropriate sling for the child.
3. Follow manufacturer's directions for applying the sling.
4. Attach sling to floor-based patient lift and activate it to raise patient out of the playpen.

Helpful Hints: Special Tips for Measuring for Pediatric Slings

Patient-lifting devices are needed to transfer physically dependent pediatric patients from bed to chair. Use the algorithm for patient transfers with the following special caveat: make special effort to ensure the sling is appropriate. For a pediatric sling, measure the width across buttocks and lower trunk, then measure the height of trunk. As with all patient-lifting equipment, follow manufacturer instructions.

7.8

Transferring the child from playpen to chair with a mechanical floor lift

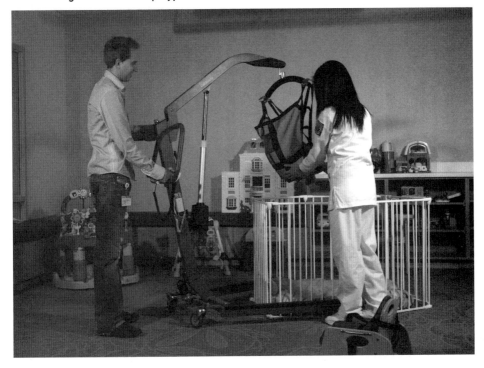

Case Study 7-1

You are caring for a teenage male who has sustained a traumatic brain injury and is in a low-level coma. Unfortunately, this teen has also suffered a C4-level spinal cord injury. He is sharing a room with one other patient. Both these teens have lots of needed equipment in the room, thus limited space for movement and transfers. The teen under your care weighs 160 lbs (72.7 kg).

Discussion Questions

1. What is the safe best practice in providing a transfer of this teen from his bed to a stretcher for his morning care in the tub room?
2. What has to happen first with the equipment and clutter in the patient room?
3. What is the best type of lifting equipment to be used, considering the large amount of patient equipment in the room?
4. How many caregivers are needed to move this patient?

Post-Test Questions

7-1. How many kilograms should a pediatric patient weigh to trigger the use of lifting equipment?
   a. 16
   b. 20
   c. 25
   d. 26

7-2. How many caregivers are needed to lift an uncooperative pediatric patient who weighs 50 kg?
   a. One
   b. Two
   c. Three
   d. Four

7-3. When you are lifting a comatose male teenager (adult size, adult weight, and adult height) from bed to wheelchair, what should you do?
   a. Use appropriate adult algorithm for this transfer.
   b. Use pediatric algorithm.
   c. Allow patient to remain in bed.
   d. None of the above.

7-4. If a child weighs more than 30 kg and needs to be lifted from the floor, which of the following is most appropriate?
   a. Use a floor-based patient lift.
   b. Lift the child alone.
   c. Lift the child with two caregivers.
   d. None of the above.

7-5. You are caring for a 12-year-old boy who needs to be transferred to his wheelchair from his bed. You are unable to locate the appropriate size of sling for the child. What is the first thing that you should do?
   a. Use whatever sling is available on the unit.
   b. Manually lift him into his wheelchair.
   c. Obtain a sling that is the proper size for the child.
   d. None of the above.

7-6. You are a new caregiver working in the adolescent unit. During the hospital orientation, you are educated on the adult safe-lifting equipment available. One of your patients requires a lift to get him out of bed. The equipment on the pediatric floor is different from the one you have been trained on. What do you do?
   a. Inform your charge caregiver that you have not been trained on this piece of equipment.
   b. Do the lift with the unfamiliar equipment.
   c. Ask a coworker to complete the lift until you receive training.
   d. Both *a* and *c* are correct.

7-7. The best way to evaluate the size of a sling for a patient in pediatrics is to:
   a. Use an adult small size
   b. Measure the child as per manufacturer's protocol
   c. Assume it is safe to manually lift children
   d. All of the above

References

Department of Veterans Affairs (VHA) VISN 8 Patient Safety Center of Inquiry. (2001). *Patient care ergonomic resource guide: Safe patient handling and movement.* Retrieved April 5, 2008, from http://www.visn8.med.va.gov/patientsafetycenter/safePtHandling/default.asp

Waters, T. (2007). When is it safe to manually lift a patient? The Revised NIOSH Lifting Equation provides support for recommended weight limits. *American Journal of Nursing, 107*(8), 53–58.

Additional Reading

American Nurses Association. (2003). Handle With Care®: The American Nurses Association's campaign to address work-related musculoskeletal disorders. Retrieved February, 23, 2008, from http://nursingworld.org/MainMenuCategories/ANAMarketplace/ANAPeriodicals/OJIN/TableofContents/Volume92004/Number3September30/HandleWithCare.aspx

American Nurses Association. (2003). Position statement on elimination of manual patient handling to prevent work-related musculoskeletal disorders. Silver Spring, MD: Author.

Burke, J. P. (2003). Infection control: A problem for patient safety. *New England Journal of Medicine, 348*(7), 651–656.

Department of Veterans Affairs (VHA) VISN 8 Patient Safety Center of Inquiry. (2005). Assessment criteria and care plan and standard safe patient handling and movement algorithms. Retrieved on April 6, 2008 from http://www.visn8.med.va.gov/visn8/patientsafetycenter/safePtHandling/default.asp

Evanoff, B., Wolf, L., Aton, E., Canos, J., & Collins, J. (2003). Reduction in injury rates in nursing personnel through introduction of mechanical lifts in the workplace. *American Journal of Industrial Medicine, 44*(5), 4510–457.

Hignett, S., Crumpton, E., Ruszala, S., Alexander, P., Fray, M., & Fletcher, B. (2003). Evidence-based patient handling: Systemic review. *Nursing Standard, 17*(33), 33–36.

Keir, P. J., & MacDonell, C. W. (2004). Muscle activity during patient transfers: A preliminary study on the influence of lift assists and experience. *Ergonomics, 47*(3), 296–306.

Menzel, N., Hughes, N., Waters, T., Shores, L., Nelson, A. (2007). Preventing musculoskeletal disorders in nurses: A safe patient handling curriculum module for nursing schools. *Nurse Educator, 32*(3), 130–135.

Nelson, A. L. (Ed.). (2006). *Handle with care: A practice guide for safe patient handling and movement.* New York: Springer.

Nelson, A., Fragala, G., & Menzel, N. (2003). Myths and facts about back injuries in nursing. *American Journal of Nursing, 103*(2), 32–41.

Nelson, A., Hughes, N., Waters, T., Hagan, P., Menzel, N., Powell-Cope, G., Sedlak, C., & Thompson, V. (2007). Effectiveness of an evidence-based curriculum module in nursing schools targeting safe patient handling and movement. *International Journal of Nursing Education Scholarship, 4*(1), 26.

Nelson, A., Lloyd, J., Gross, C., & Menzel, N. (2001). *Redesigning patient handling tasks to prevent nursing back injuries.* Research Report #95-1502 to Veterans Health Administration.

Nelson, A., Lloyd, J., Menzel, N., & Gross, C. (2003). Preventing nursing back injuries: Redesigning patient handling tasks. *The American Association of Occupational Health Nurses Journal, 51*(3), 126–34.

Nelson, A., & Owen, B. (2003). Safe patient handling movement. *American Journal of Nursing, 103*(3) 32–44.

Nelson, A., Owen, B., Lloyd, J. D., Fragala, G., Matz, M.W., Amato, M., Bowers, J., Moss-Cureton, S., Ramser, G., & Lentz, K. (2003). Safe patient handling and movement. Preventing back injury among nurses requires careful selection of the safest equipment and techniques. *American Journal of Nursing, 103*(3), 32–44.

Nelson, A., & Baptiste, A. S. (2004). Evidence-based practices for safe patient handling and movement. *Online Journal of Issues in Nursing, 9*(3), Manuscript 3, 1–26.

NIOSH Publication No. 2006-117. (2006). Safe lifting and movement of nursing home residents. Retrieved February 23, 2008, from http://www.cdc.gov/niosh/docs/2006-117/.html

Rush, A. (2004). Assessing clients for the correct hoist or sling: A practical guide. *International Journal of Therapy and Rehabilitation, 11*(4), 179–182.

Smith, L., Weinel, D., Doloresco, L., & Lloyd, J. (2002). A clinical evaluation of ceiling lifts: Lifting and transfer technology for the future. *SCI Nursing, 19*(2), 75–77.

Swain, J., Pufahl, E. R., & Williamson, G. (2003). Do they practice what we teach? A survey of manual handling practice amongst student nurses. *Journal of Clinical Nursing, 12*(2), 297–306.

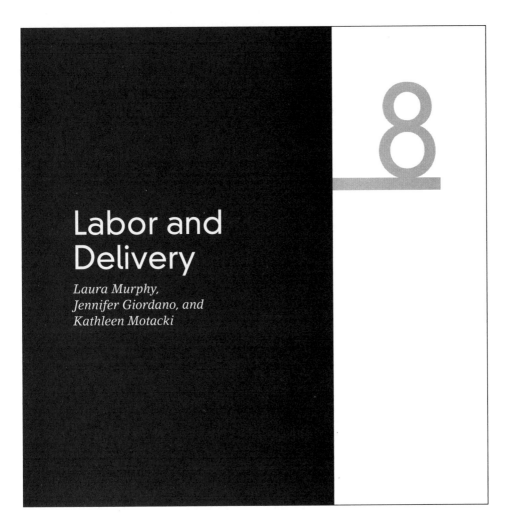

8

Labor and Delivery

*Laura Murphy,
Jennifer Giordano, and
Kathleen Motacki*

Description of Setting/Unique Challenges

Labor-and-delivery settings are often fast paced and unpredictable, which increases the risk of musculoskeletal injuries associated with patient handling. Although many of the patients in labor-and-delivery settings are alert and able to follow directions, a large number receive epidural medications, which can interfere with the ability to cooperate with repositioning. The purpose of this chapter is to identify high-risk patient-practical solutions applicable to labor-and-delivery units. When referring to the patient, it is the laboring patient.

High-Risk Tasks

Four high-risk patient-handling tasks have been identified in this specialty area of nursing:

1. Repositioning during labor
2. Positioning patient for epidural
3. Repositioning patient to foot of bed in preparation for delivery
4. Holding legs of patient for delivery

Objectives

1. Describe the unique challenges associated with safe patient handling in labor-and-delivery units.
2. Identify high-risk patient-handling tasks in labor-and-delivery units.

Pre-Test Questions

8-1. What is the safest way to move a patient to the end of the bed in preparation for delivery?
   a. With at least two caregivers, manually pull the laboring patient down to end of the bed.
   b. Use a friction-reducing device (FRD) and at least two caregivers.
   c. One person can secure the laboring patient's feet and gently pull the laboring patient to the end of the bed.
   d. Always have the patient perform this task by herself to promote independence.

8-2. What is the best approach for lateral transfer of a patient who has had an epidural block?
   a. Follow the algorithm for lateral transfers presented under common patient-transfer tasks.
   b. Always have the patient position herself.
   c. Enlist help of other staff to manually transfer the patient.
   d. Use the labor algorithm.

8-3. When preparing to reposition a patient during labor, what is the first step?
   a. Use the appropriate algorithm.
   b. Assess the strength of the caregiver.
   c. Check number of staff available to help.
   d. Assess the patient.

8-4. What is the best approach for holding a patient's legs during delivery?
   a. One caregiver and a patient lift with appropriate limb-lift sling
   b. Two caregivers; one to manually hold each limb
   c. One caregiver and stirrups
   d. Two or more caregivers and an FRD

8-5. How would instructing the patient on repositioning be beneficial?
   a. It would decrease the injury risk to the caregiver.
   b. It would make the patient's labor longer.
   c. It would decrease patient's anxiety.
   d. It would include the friends and family in the labor process.

General Directions for All Tasks

1. Complete *Assessment Criteria and Care Plan* for patient. Key assessment factors include physical ability to assist, ability to follow instructions, and cooperation. *Note: Weight and height may trigger use of bariatric algorithms.*

2. Assess the patient and review the high-risk patient-handling task to be performed and determine the number of caregivers, types of equipment, and techniques for performing each high risk patient-handling task safely. If no algorithm exists, use the techniques described in this book to guide practice.

3. Check the weight capacity of the equipment to be sure it is able to handle the patient's weight.

4. Remove obstacles to performing the patient-handling tasks. Obstacles include too little room to maneuver the equipment, equipment stored on the floor posing a stumbling hazard, or inability to perform the activity without threats to patient dignity (e.g., lack of privacy). You may need to remove chairs or bed tables, separate beds, move floor-based equipment, and ask visitors to leave.

5. Make sure selected equipment is in good working order. If the equipment is battery operated, check that the battery is charged. Verify that the appropriate slings and attachments are available. Review safe operation of the equipment, including location of emergency buttons or manual controls in the event of a power failure.

6. Ensure sufficient caregivers are available to help, as specified in the algorithm.

7. Make sure beds are adjusted to caregiver's waist/elbow height before performing bed-related patient-handling tasks.

8. Explain the procedure to the patient and assisting caregivers.

9. Wear gloves according to proper infection control practices and facility policies.

Side-to-Side Repositioning During Labor Using FRDs

Description of Task and Associated Risks

Constant patient repositioning from side to side during labor involves the caregiver-risk factors of lifting heavy loads, twisting, awkward postures, and frequency. Patient-risk factors include lifting heavy loads and awkward postures. When a patient goes into labor, she may have reached a bariatric weight. Frequent position changes are necessary to promote patient comfort and maintain the infant's heart rate.

View Video 2.7: Bed Repositioning With FRD for the Partially Dependent Patient (Chapter 2)

Patient Abilities

■ Physically unable to assist or uncooperative

Resources Required

■ Friction-reducing device (FRD)
■ Two caregivers

Technique 8-1

1. Follow the same guidelines as in chapter 2, Technique 2-8.
2. Use one caregiver to position fetal monitor wires and pillows. The caregiver must also give the patient verbal cues for position change.
3. With the use of the FRD, the caregivers can assist the patient to reposition side to side during labor. Place pillows behind laboring patient's back to maintain side-lying position.

Repositioning in Bed Using Ceiling-Mounted Patient Lift

Description of Task and Associated Risks

Caregivers must frequently reposition patients in bed for a number of reasons, including promoting patient comfort and improving fetal circulation; therefore, preventing a decrease in fetal heart rate.

Refer to Appendix A, Algorithm 4. This algorithm provides various methods for repositioning the patient in bed using equipment, such as FRDs or full body sling lifts, depending on patient abilities. The methods of choice have many patient variables including size, weight, and the number of caregivers available to assist. The caregiver must also consider the patient's pain, level of fatigue, and ability to cooperate. There are several tips included in the algorithm to assist the caregivers. The caregiver must also ensure that other key factors are being addressed such as the bed height, body postures, and communication between all participants during the maneuvers. When the patients can assist, coach them to use the side rails and overhead repositioning bars.

Patient Abilities

■ Unable to assist

Resources Required

■ Ceiling-mounted patient lift
■ Supine total-body sling, hammock sling, or repositioning sling
■ Two or more caregivers
■ Pillows to sustain patient in side-lying position

The ceiling-mounted patient lift and repositioning sling are the preferred equipment combination for this task.

Helpful Hint

After a few bed repositions, the repositioning sling needs to be relocated in proper position under the patient. In this patient-care setting, replace the sling frequently because of soiling from the patient's body fluids. Position the new sling while the patient is suspended in the lift in the original sling.

Technique 8-2

1. Follow *General Directions for All Tasks*.
2. Apply sling using side-to-side rolling technique. Position top of sling under patient's head. If sling is already in place, assess if current position is appropriate for use.
3. To attach sling to lift and lower head of bed to semi-Fowler position if patient can tolerate.
4. Ensure a pillow is positioned under the patient's head and shoulders. Position sling attachment bar lengthwise to patient.
5. Attach loop sling straps to overhead attachment bar on lift. Ensure they are attached evenly and equally distributed at each end of the attachment bar. The loops to be attached should be each side of sling at the head, shoulders, hips, and lower legs.

Helpful Hint

Floor-based patient lifts are not recommended for use in the labor-and-delivery room due to the high number of health care workers present. When there is a high-risk delivery, there is one team for the patient and one team for the baby.

6. Using the operational controls, raise patient off the bed 2–3 inches. Assess patient tolerance and weight distribution in the sling.
7. Slide the ceiling-mounted patient lift toward the head of the bed using the track; gently guide patient's body, lightly pushing sling to desirable position.
8. If the patient is to be side-lying, then also move the patient to the side of the bed using the track.
9. Using the controls, lower patient to bed.
10. Remove straps from sling, maintaining straps on one side of lift, which will assist the patient to turn side-lying. Maintain sling bar lengthwise to patient.
11. Using the controls, raise the lift slightly using the up button; this will turn the patient onto her side.
12. Position pillows for patient comfort and to maintain position.
13. Lower lift and remove sling straps.
14. Determine whether sling can be left under patient, considering the patient will be turning frequently while in labor.
15. Do not leave ceiling-mounted patient lift hanging over the patient.

8.1

Attaching the sling to the ceiling lift

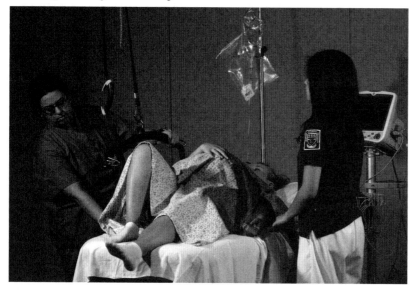

Positioning the Patient in Bed for Epidural: Side Lying Position Using Ceiling-Mounted Patient Lift

Description of Task and Associated Risks

View Video 8.1: Side to Side Patient Reposition for Epidural

View Video 8.2: Repositioning Patient on Side Using Repositioning Sling

Usually when the patient is about to receive an epidural, she is in a great deal of pain and, at times, unable to assist with position changes. The patient must be in proper position for the anesthesiologist to help ensure a safe procedure. The caregiver risks are awkward postures, twisting movements, and long duration of positions.

Patient Abilities

- Physically unable to assist or uncooperative

Resources Required

- Ceiling-mounted patient lift with repositioning sling
- One caregiver using ceiling-mounted patient lift with repositioning; two caregivers if the patient is uncooperative

Technique 8-3

1. Follow *General Directions for All Tasks*.
2. Follow same procedure as for repositioning laboring patient in bed using ceiling-mounted patient lift.
3. Once the patient is in proper position, remove sling so the epidural can be administered by the anesthesiologist.

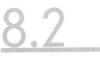

Repositioning patient on side using repositioning sling

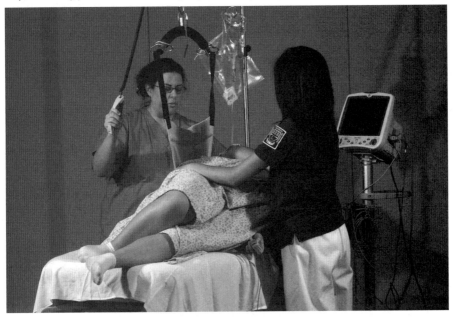

Positioning the Patient for Epidural: Seated Position

Description of Task and Associated Risks

If the anesthesiologist requests that the patient be placed in the seated position for an epidural, the best method is to use an FRD. The caregiver risks are moving heavy loads and awkward positions. Once the patient has received an epidural block, positioning the patient is more of a challenge because the patient can no longer assist with positioning and repositioning.

Patient Abilities

■ Partially able to assist

Resources Required

■ One–two FRDs, depending on patient's ability to assist
■ One–three caregivers for a patient ≤ 200 lbs or three or more caregivers if patient >200 lbs

Technique 8-4

1. Follow *General Directions for All Tasks.*
2. Position bed flat or with head slightly elevated.
3. Ask or assist the patient to roll from side to side to place the FRDs underneath patient's buttocks.
4. Once the FRD is under the patient's buttocks, Caregiver "A" will assist by turning patient's legs to the right so that the feet are on a chair or stool.
5. Caregiver "B" will assist by turning patient's hips to the right as Caregiver "A" is turning legs.
6. Assist laboring patient to hold onto chair with head down and back in hunched-over position during administration of epidural.
7. The FRD will remain in place until after the procedure is performed.
8. The caregivers will then reverse the procedure so the patient can return to supine position.

8.3

Repositioning the patient for epidural: seated position

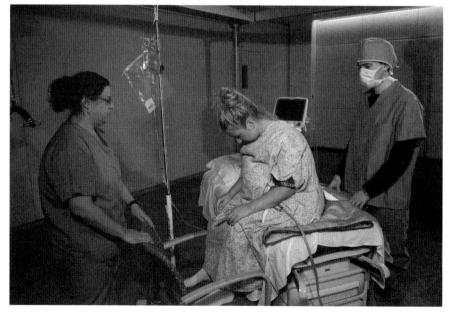

Repositioning Patient to Foot of the Bed in Preparation for Delivery

Description of Task and Associated Risks

Once the physician determines that the patient is ready for delivery, the patient must be positioned with the buttocks at the end of the delivery table. Usually the patient has had an epidural and is unable to assist. The risk factors to the caregivers are lifting heavy loads and prolonged positions.

Patient Abilities

- Physically unable to assist or uncooperative

Resources Required

- Ceiling-mounted lift
- Supine total body sling, hammock sling, or repositioning sling
- Two or more caregivers, depending on patient weight

The ceiling-mounted patient lift and repositioning sling are the preferred equipment combination for this task.

Technique 8-5

1. Follow *General Directions for All Tasks*.
2. Apply sling using side-to-side rolling technique. Position top of sling under patient's head.
3. To attach sling to lift, lower head of bed flat if patient can tolerate.
4. Ensure a pillow is positioned under the patient's head and shoulders. Position sling attachment bar lengthwise to patient.
5. Attach loop sling straps to overhead attachment bar on lift. Ensure they are attached evenly and equally distributed at each end of the attachment bar. The loops to be attached should be at each side of sling at the head, shoulders, hips, and lower legs.
6. Using the operational controls, raise patient off the bed 2–3 inches. Assess patient tolerance and weight distribution in the sling.
7. Slide the ceiling-mounted patient lift toward the end of the bed using the track; gently guide patient's body, lightly pushing sling to desirable position.
8. Using the controls, lower patient to bed.
9. Lower lift and remove sling straps.
10. Determine whether sling can be left under patient, considering contraindications of large amounts of bodily fluids during delivery of baby.
11. Do not leave ceiling-mounted patient lift hanging over the patient.
12. Place patient's feet in stirrups.

8.4

Positioning for delivery

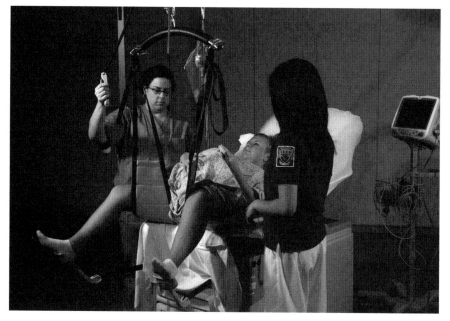

Repositioning Patient to End of Delivery Table Using FRDs

Description of Task and Associated Risks

Once the patient is ready for delivery of the baby, she must slide down to the end of the delivery table.

Refer to Appendix A, Algorithm 4. This algorithm provides various methods to reposition the patient in bed using equipment, such as FRDs or full-body sling lift, depending on patient abilities. The methods of choice have many patient variables including size, weight, and the number of caregivers available to assist while the mother is laboring. The caregiver must consider the patient's pain, level of fatigue, and ability to cooperate. There are several tips included in the algorithm to assist the caregivers. The caregiver must also ensure that other key factors are being addressed such as the bed height, body postures, and communication between all participants during the maneuvers. When the patient can assist, clear instructions must be given at all times.

Patient Abilities

■ Unable to assist

Resources Required

- One–two FRDs, depending on patient's ability to assist
- One–three caregivers for a patient ≤ 200 lbs, or three or more caregivers if patient >200 lbs

Technique 8-6

1. Follow *General Directions for All Tasks*.
2. Position delivery table at elbow level to move patient down in bed.
3. Assist the patient to roll from side to side to place the FRDs underneath patient's back and buttocks.
4. Complete the following steps:
   a. One caregiver on each side of the patient should slide patient down to desired place on delivery table. Each caregiver grips (palms up, with wrist rotation neutral if possible) the handles or edge of the uppermost FRD.
   b. Repeat procedure until patient has reached desired position on table.
   c. With back straight and a wide base of support, flex knees and hips, and keep elbows close to sides.
   d. One designated caregiver will communicate that the movement will begin on the three count, and then count to three.
   e. Shift weight onto the leg closest to the foot of the table while sliding the patient toward the foot of the table using the upper FRD. Remember, do not twist.

8.5

Two caregivers using FRD to reposition laboring patient on delivery table in preparation for delivery

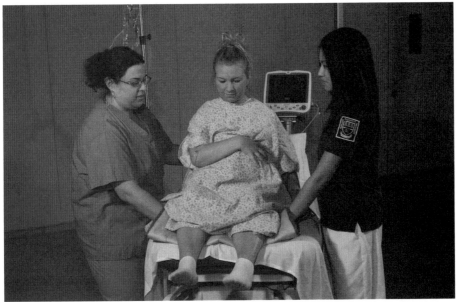

Holding Legs of Patient for Delivery

Description of Task and Associated Risks

Once the patient's buttocks are in the proper position at the bottom of the delivery table, the patient's legs must be elevated for the delivery. By this time the patient has had an epidural and is unable to assist with lower-body movements. Because limb lifting for long periods of time is a high-risk task, the patient's legs should be maintained in position using the limb-lifting slings. (Refer to positioning and holding legs for access to perineum in critical care chapter.)

View Video 5.1: Patient Transport with Power Drive Bed (Chapter 5)

Patient Abilities

- Physically unable to assist or uncooperative

Resources Required

- Ceiling-mounted patient lift and limb sling
- One caregiver using ceiling-mounted patient lift
- Two caregivers if the patient is uncooperative

Technique 8-7

1. Follow *General Directions for All Tasks.*
2. See Technique 5-1 in chapter 5 for use of limb-lifting sling.
3. Place laboring patient's feet in stirrups.

Helpful Hint

If the patient must be transported in a bed to the delivery room for an emergency delivery or a cesarean section, use a bed mover due to the high forces required to move heavy beds occupied by a patient.
See chapter 5, Critical Care

4. Place limb sling under laboring patient's legs.
5. Attach sling to ceiling-mounted lift. (Floor lift not recommended in delivery room. The ceiling-mounted lift and repositioning sling are the preferred equipment combination for this task. Although a floor-based patient lift can be used to perform these tasks, this equipment can get in the way because of the number of care providers present.)
6. Raise lift to desired height.
7. As lift is being raised, both of laboring patient's thighs will go into delivery position. See Chapter 5, Figures 5.1 and 5.2.
8. Continue with above until laboring patient is in proper position for delivery.
9. Reposition stirrups so that laboring patient is in proper position for delivery.

Case Study 8-1

You are the nurse admitting a 32-year-old Gravida 1, Para 0, laboring patient. She is contracting every 5–7 minutes, with each contraction lasting 30–60 seconds. When examined, her membranes are intact and she is 4 cm dilated, 70% effaced, station -3. She is admitted and immediately requests an epidural. The patient is constantly reassessed while in labor. Approximately 6 hours after the patient's admittance, the nurse finds the patient to be fully dilated, station 0. The patient needs to begin pushing, and the nurse must position her for the delivery.

Discussion Questions:

1. What is the most important assessment factor in determining how to safely reposition this patient?
2. Practice explaining the procedure used to reposition the laboring patient to the foot of the bed in preparation for delivery.
3. What is the first step in positioning the laboring patient for the delivery?
4. What types of equipment and how many caregivers are needed to perform this task safely?
5. If the equipment you need is being used for another patient, what is the best action to take?

Post-Test Questions

8-1. What is the safest way to move a patient to the end of the bed in preparation for delivery?
   a. With at least two caregivers, manually pull the laboring patient down to end of the bed.
   b. Use a friction-reducing device (FRD) and at least two caregivers.
   c. One person can secure the laboring patient's feet and gently pull the laboring patient to the end of the bed.
   d. Always have the patient perform this task by herself to promote independence.
8-2. What is the best approach for lateral transfer of a patient who has had an epidural block?
   a. Follow the algorithm for lateral transfers presented under common patient-transfer tasks.
   b. Always have the patient position herself.
   c. Enlist help of other staff to manually transfer the patient.
   d. Use the labor algorithm.
8-3. When preparing to reposition a patient during labor, what is the first step?
   a. Use the appropriate algorithm.
   b. Assess the strength of the caregiver.
   c. Check number of staff available to help.
   d. Assess the patient.
8-4. What is the best approach for holding a patient's legs during delivery?
   a. One caregiver and a patient lift with appropriate limb-lift sling
   b. Two caregivers; one to manually hold each limb

    c. One caregiver and stirrups

    d. Two or more caregivers and an FRD

8-5. How would instructing the patient on repositioning be beneficial?

    a. It would decrease the injury risk to the caregiver.

    b. It would make the patient's labor longer.

    c. It would decrease patient's anxiety.

    d. It would include the friends and family in the labor process.

Additional Reading

Aiken, L. H., Clarke, S.P., Sloane, D. M., Sochalski, J., & Silber, J. H. (2002). Hospital nurse staffing and patient mortality, nurse burnout, and job dissatisfaction. *Journal of the American Medical Association, 288,* 1987–1993.

Brown, J. G., Trinkoff, A., Rempher, K., McPhaul, K., Brady, B., Lipscomb, J., et al. (2005). Nurses' inclination to report work-related injuries: Organizational, work-group, and individual factors associated with reporting. *AAOHN Journal, 53*(5), 213–217.

Hignett, S., Crompton, E., Ruszala, S., Alexander, P., Fray, M., & Fletcher, B. (2003). *Evidence-based patient handling: Tasks, equipment and interventions.* New York: Routledge.

Menzel, N. N. (2004). Back pain prevalence in nursing personnel: Measurement issues. *AAOHN Journal, 52*(2), 54–65.

Nelson, A. L. (Ed.). (2006). *Safe patient handling and movement: A practical guide for health care professionals.* New York: Springer.

Nelson, A. L., & Fragala, G. (2004). Equipment for safe patient handling and movement. In W. Charney & A. Hudson (Eds.), *Back injury among healthcare workers* (pp. 121–135). Washington, DC: Lewis Publishers.

Nelson, A. L., Lloyd, J., Menzel, N., & Gross, C. (2003). Preventing nursing back injuries: Redesigning patient handling tasks. *AAOHN Journal, 51*(3), 126–134.

Owen, B., & Garg, A. (1993). Back stress isn't part of the job. *American Journal of Nursing, 93*(2), 48–51.

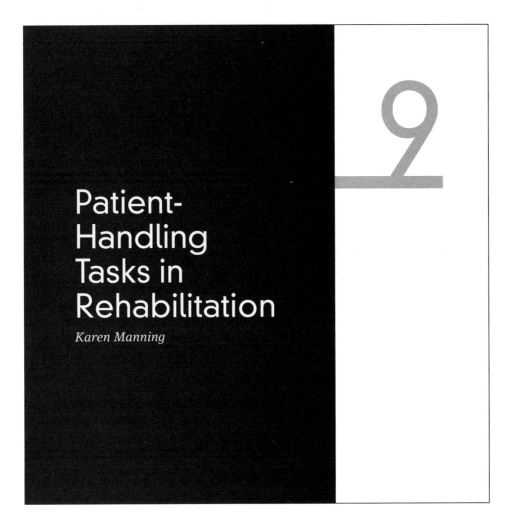

Patient-Handling Tasks in Rehabilitation

Karen Manning

Description of Setting

The purpose of rehabilitation is to assist individuals affected by chronic illness or physical disability to reach their fullest potential and adapt to an altered lifestyle. Successful rehabilitation is contingent on a team approach in which each team member brings a unique perspective and individual expertise but also works with the patient/family to achieve optimal outcomes. The delivery of care in rehabilitation presents challenges to the direct health care provider, who must compensate for mobility and self-care deficits. Functional movement, muscle activation, and sensory stimulation play an essential role in maximizing functional ability. Patient-handling tasks, such as transfers, positioning, lifting, ambulation, and activities of daily living are therapeutically aimed to increase endurance, make joints less stiff, strengthen muscles, reduce pain, and improve coordination and balance.

Unique Challenges to Providing Safe Patient Handling in this Setting

Many patient-handling tasks in rehabilitation are performed at high risk to the caregivers, resulting in musculoskeletal injuries. A critical challenge in rehabilitation is to create safe working environments for caregivers that do not compromise rehabilitation goals for the patient. Goals for patients include improving functional levels and promoting independence. Initial resistance to use of patient handling in rehabilitation was based on concerns that the devices would "make the patient more dependent" or somehow delay rehabilitation progress. To address these concerns, Dr. Audrey Nelson (an editor of this book) led an interdisciplinary task force, which included representation from the American Physical Therapy Association (APTA), the Association of Rehabilitation Nurses (ARN), and the Veterans Hospital Administration (VHA). This group published a white paper addressing the need for a description of safe patient handling in a rehabilitation setting, with a dual emphasis on protection of caregiver and patient related to patient-handling tasks (Nelson et al., 2005). The paper recommends the development of policies and procedures for "therapeutic use" of patient-handling equipment and for research to identify therapeutic ways to use patient-handling equipment. To ensure safety for all, nurses and therapists must work together to integrate patient-handling equipment with the patient's functional ability, discuss how the patient can assist with the activity, and implement a succession of equipment types (from dependent lifts to assistive equipment) as the patient progresses in the rehabilitation program.

High-Risk Tasks

Rehabilitation involves patient handling and movement of persons with disabilities. Several high-risk tasks related to patient transfers are described in other chapters and will not be repeated here. The high-risk tasks that have been identified for rehabilitation settings are listed below:

- Neurogenic bowel care: supine position
- Neurogenic bowel care: seated position
- Ambulating a patient at risk for falls
- Bathing/showering out of bed
- Special transfer approach for a patient with a lower-limb amputation

Objectives

1. Describe the unique challenges associated with safe patient handling in rehabilitation patient populations.
2. Identify high-risk patient-handling tasks on rehabilitation units.
3. Delineate the number of caregivers, types of equipment, and techniques for performing each high-risk patient-handling task safely.

Pre-Test Questions

9-1. Which of the following rehabilitation tasks involves heavy lifting and awkward posture?
   a. Neurogenic bowel care for an individual with a complete C4 spinal cord injury (SCI)
   b. Transferring an individual with multiple sclerosis (MS) with lower-extremity spasticity into a shower chair
   c. Putting compression stockings on an individual with a left cerebral vascular accident (CVA)
   d. All of the above

9-2. When a caregiver performs neurogenic bowel care for a patient in bed, what factors *most* contribute to risk?
   a. Holding the body in a side-lying position to access the rectum
   b. Twisting and reaching
   c. Pulling and pushing
   d. All of the above

9-3. What are the benefits of using safe patient-handling equipment in rehabilitation?
   a. Reduce the risk of musculoskeletal injuries in the caregiver.
   b. Reduce the risk of patient falls when ambulating patients.
   c. Equipment can be selected to match patient's functional ability as the patient progresses in the rehabilitation program.
   d. All of the above.

9-4. Which type of sling is the most appropriate for a tub bath for an individual with a T5 SCI?
   a. A supine sling is most appropriate.
   b. A hygienic seated sling is most appropriate for bathing.
   c. An ambulation sling is most appropriate.
   d. It is not safe for persons with an SCI to have a tub bath.

9-5. The primary function of a special amputee sling is to:
   a. Ambulate an individual with an above-the-knee amputation in preparation for a prosthesis
   b. Support the whole body up to shoulder height and pelvis region to prevent possible slip or fall due to shift in center of gravity and imbalance
   c. Reposition an individual with a below-the-knee amputation to a prone position to allow extension of the hip and knee of the residual leg
   d. None of the above

General Directions for All Tasks

1. Complete *Assessment Criteria and Care Plan* for patient. Key assessment factors include physical ability to assist, ability to follow instructions, and cooperation. *Note: Weight and height may trigger use of bariatric algorithms.*
2. Review the algorithm for the high-risk patient-handling task to be performed and determine the number of caregivers, types of equipment, and techniques for performing each high-risk patient-handling task safely. If no algorithm exists, use the techniques described in this book to guide practice.

3. Check the weight capacity of the equipment to be sure it is able to handle the patient's weight.
4. Remove obstacles to performing the patient-handling tasks. Obstacles include too little room to maneuver the equipment, equipment stored on the floor posing a stumbling hazard, or inability to perform the activity without threats to patient dignity (e.g., lack of privacy). You may need to remove chairs or bed tables, separate beds, move floor-based equipment, and ask visitors to leave.
5. Make sure selected equipment is in good working order. If the equipment is battery operated, check that the battery is charged. Verify that the appropriate slings and attachments are available. Review safe operation of the equipment, including location of emergency buttons or manual controls for the event of a power failure.
6. Ensure sufficient caregivers are available to help, as specified in the algorithm.
7. Make sure beds are adjusted to caregiver's waist/elbow height before performing bed-related patient-handling tasks.
8. Explain the procedure to the patient and assisting caregivers.
9. Wear gloves according to proper infection-control practices and facility policies.

Neurogenic Bowel Care: Supine Position

Description of Task and Associated Risks

Inpatient rehabilitation units have a high proportion of patients requiring assistance with activities of daily living, including neurogenic bowel care. Neurogenic bowel is the loss of normal bowel function caused by damage to part of the nervous system (American Association of Spinal Cord Injury Nurses, 2007). The sitting position on a toilet or commode is preferred so that gravity can assist bowel emptying. Orthostatic hypotension, pressure ulcers, skin grafts, and other conditions may prevent a sitting position, requiring a left-side-lying position in bed. Due to sensory deficits and high risk for pressure ulcers, no bedpan is used during this procedure. Many patients are able to perform this task independently despite paralysis; the caregiver's role may be to assist with setup if needed. Caregiver risk associated with performing bowel care includes sustained awkward position, as well as excessive reaching and twisting.

Patient Abilities

■ Unable to assist due to limited hand function or cognitive deficits

Resources Needed

■ Friction-reducing devices (FRDs) or ceiling-mounted patient lift with supine repositioning sling. The ceiling-mounted patient lift and repositioning sling are the preferred equipment combination for this task. The repositioning sling allows access to patient's skin for inspection, treatment, and bowel care, as seen in Figure 9.1.

- Depending on the patient's capabilities, bed-repositioning poles may also be of benefit for patient to assist himself/herself.
- This task has two parts:
  1. For positioning the patient in preparation for the bowel-care procedure:
     - Two caregivers are needed to reposition patient when using an FRD.
     - One caregiver is needed when using a ceiling mounted patient lift.
  2. For performing bowel care:
     - One caregiver is needed; if the patient is uncooperative, an additional caregiver may be needed.
     - Pillows (one–three) for maintaining patient in side-lying positions during the bowel program.
     - Supplies for neurogenic bowel care.

Technique 9-1

1. Follow *General Directions for All Tasks*.
2. Position bed flat or, if possible, with head slightly down (if patient able to tolerate).
3. If using an FRD, place it underneath patient's head, shoulders, back, and legs, following Technique 3-16 (chapter 3). If using a ceiling-mounted patient lift, apply sling according to manufacturer's guidelines. Press down on the mattress and slide the small repositioning sling under patient's lower back. A side-to-side rolling technique and one additional caregiver may be required; if patient is able to assist, instruct patient to assist with turning side to side.
4. For left-side repositioning using an FRD, complete the following steps:
   a. Caregiver "A" (facing the direction the patient will face) will pull slightly up and toward himself or herself on the FRD to tip the patient onto his/her left side.
   b. Caregiver "B" will assist by placing one hand on the patient's right shoulder and one on the patient's right hip. Caregiver "B" will push slightly, moving the patient away.
   c. Caregiver "B" will hold the patient on the left side by taking the FRD from the far side of the bed and tipping the patient toward "B" and holding him or her on the left side. Meanwhile, "A" will insert pillows to secure the patient in the left-side-lying position, leaving the buttocks exposed.
   d. Remove the FRD.
5. For left-side positioning when using a ceiling-mounted patient lift, ensure a pillow is positioned under the patient's head and shoulders.
   a. Position sling attachment bar lengthwise to patient.
   b. Attach right side of loop sling straps to overhead attachment bar on ceiling-mounted patient lift and attach the left side to the bed frame, which will assist the patient to turn onto his or her left side. Maintain sling bar lengthwise to patient.
   c. Using the controls, raise the lift slightly using the up button; this will turn the patient onto left side.
   d. Position pillows for patient comfort and to maintain position, leaving buttocks exposed.
   e. Lower lift and remove sling straps.
   f. Leave sling under patient until bowel program is completed.

6. Place one or two incontinence pads under the patient's buttocks.
7. Begin the bowel program.
8. Lower the height of the bed for waiting periods for digital or chemical stimulation, and then readjust to the level of the caregiver's waist/elbow height if digital stimulation is repeated.
9. If using ceiling-mounted patient lift, reattach right side of loop sling straps to overhead bar on ceiling lift and use controls to lift to turn patient farther onto left side for cleaning buttocks.
   a. Lower lift and remove sling straps, leaving patient on left side.
   b. Roll sling and incontinence pad under patient and assist patient to a back-lying position.
   c. Turn patient on right side with the correct number of people to clean right side of buttocks, and remove sling and incontinence pad.
   d. Lift and move device so that it is not left hanging over the patient, and store device according to manufacturer's guidelines.
   e. Note: The sling will need to be replaced when soiled.

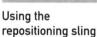

9.1

Using the repositioning sling

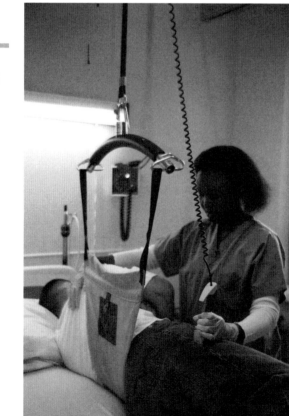

Neurogenic Bowel Care: Seated Position

Description of Task and Associated Risks

Inpatient rehabilitation units have a high proportion of patients requiring assistance with activities of daily living, including neurogenic bowel care. Neurogenic bowel is the loss of normal bowel function caused by damage to part of the nervous system (American Association of Spinal Cord Injury Nurses, 2007). The sitting position on a toilet or commode is preferred so that gravity can assist bowel emptying. Orthostatic hypotension, pressure ulcers, skin grafts, and other conditions may prevent a sitting position, requiring a left-side-lying position in bed. Due to sensory deficits and high risk of pressure ulcers, no bedpan is used during this procedure. Many patients are able to perform this task independently despite paralysis; the caregiver's role may be to assist with setup if needed. Algorithm 4 (discussed in chapter 2) provides various methods for repositioning the patient in bed. Caregiver risk associated with performing bowel care includes sustained awkward position, as well as excessive reaching, bending, and twisting.

> View Video 9.1: Neurogenic Bowel Care (Seated)

Patient Abilities

- Unable to assist due to limited hand function or cognitive deficits.

Resources Needed

- Ceiling-mounted or floor-based patient lift and seated hygiene sling. The hygiene sling exposes the buttocks; see Figure 9.2.
- Bedside commode or wheeled commode/shower chair that fits over a standard toilet (not needed if ceiling-mounted patient lift tracks extend from bedside area to bathroom, allowing for direct transfer to toilet). Consider a reclining commode chair if the patient has postural hypotension and/or poor trunk control.
- Depending on the patient's capabilities, bed-repositioning poles may also be of benefit for patient to assist.
- This task has two parts:
  1. One caregiver is needed for positioning the patient in preparation for the bowel care procedure when using a patient lift. If the patient is uncooperative, an additional caregiver may be needed.
  2. One caregiver is needed for performing bowel care. If the patient is uncooperative, an additional caregiver may be needed.
- Supplies for neurogenic bowel care.

9.2

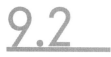

The hygiene sling

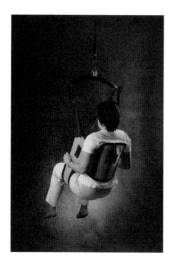

Technique 9-2

1. Follow *General Directions for All Tasks*.
2. Move commode next to bed, if using a ceiling-mounted patient lift with tracking that does not go into bathroom.
3. Select the appropriate sling for toileting.
4. To attach sling to lift, lower head of bed flat if patient can tolerate.
5. Ensure a pillow is positioned under the patient's head and shoulders.
6. Apply sling using side-to-side rolling technique and right number of people or, if patient is able to assist with upper extremities, instruct patient to assist with turning side to side. If sling is already in place, assess whether current sling position is appropriate for use. After placing sling under patient, leave patient on left side.
7. Place one or two incontinence pads under patient's buttocks.
8. Leave sling under patient until transfer to commode or toilet.
9. Attach sling to overhead attachment bar and activate motor to raise patient off the bed's surface.
10. Use manual or powered traverse to position patient over commode or toilet, then lower the patient until contact is made.
11. Lower lift and remove sling straps.
12. Leave the sling in position during bowel program (15–20 minutes).
13. If the patient is unable to lean forward for repeated digital stimulation or if twisting, bending, and awkward posture are involved, then reattach the straps to overhead attachment bar and activate motor to raise patient off the toilet for digital stimulation. Use a rolling stool to prevent awkward posture. Repeat until bowel program is completed.
14. Reattach straps to overhead attachment bar when bowel program is completed and activate motor to raise patient off commode or toilet. Clean patient's buttocks and return patient to bed or wheelchair.
15. Lower lift and remove sling straps.
16. Lift and move device so that it is not left hanging over the patient, and then store device according to manufacturer's guideline.

Ambulating a Patient at Risk for Falling

Description of Task and Associated Risks

Efforts to contain rising health care costs and to provide quality care have led to fall-preventive programs (Evitt & Quigley, 2004). Major risk factors for falls and fear of falling overlap significantly (Friedman, Munoz, West, Rubin, & Fried, 2002). Patients at risk of falling or fear of falling can benefit from a prevention program and the use of safe patient-handling equipment. Supported walking vests/systems allow patients with high risk for falls to practice gait and balance activities safety with the security of a ceiling lift or floor-based mobility lift. Risks to the caregiver include lifting heavy weights, reaching, and awkward postures. Risks to the patient include skin shearing.

> View Video 9.2: Ambulating a Patient at Risk for Falls, Using a Ceiling-Mounted Patient Lift

Patient Abilities

- Able to bear weight
- Cooperative and able to follow instructions
- Low endurance or poor balance
- Fall risk

Resources Required

- Floor-based patient lift, sit-to-stand lift, or ceiling-mounted patient lift. These lifts can act as assistive devices for gait/walking and balance training, as well as for patients who are at risk of or afraid of falling. The base of floor-based lifts readily adjusts to the desired width and can accommodate a walker. The footrest for the sit-to-stand lift is removable to allow for ambulation. Some lifts can be equipped with armrests for support and added security. The advantages of the ceiling-mounted lift for ambulation are that there are no obstacles in the walking path and the patient feels more secure. The disadvantage is that ambulation is restricted to where there are ceiling tracks.
- Ambulation sling: There are several sling options that can be used with the lift; the caregiver must ensure the sling is appropriate for standing and ambulation. These decisions are based on the amount of support needed, as well as the comfort of the patient. It is important to select the right size. (See Sling Technology Resource Guide at http://www.visn8. med.va.gov/patiensafetycenter/safePtHandling/toolkitSlings.asp.)
- One caregiver
- Walker

Technique 9-3

1. Follow *General Directions for All Tasks*.
2. Select and inspect the appropriate ambulation sling size and type for the patient.

3. Follow manufacturer's directions for applying sling. Some slings will require the patient to be lying down, whereas other standing/ambulating slings can be applied while in a sitting position. Encourage the patient to apply sling or assist to increase patient's trunk control and upper-extremity strength.
4. If using a floor-based patient lift or sit-to-stand lift, move it so that the open end of the base encloses the patient.
5. Attach loops/clips to lift. Encourage the patient to independently attach the loops or assist to increase fine motor skills and strengthen fingers, wrists, and upper arms.

Helpful Hint

Ensure mast is lowered enough to avoid pulling on or lifting the sling during attachment to the lift.

6. For floor-based patient lifts, lock brakes before patient stands. (If using a walker, place in front of patient.)
7. Instruct patient to stand by leaning forward and pushing off with hands from the bed or chair/wheelchair. As patient stands, activate the motor lifting to keep the straps equally taut.
8. Once standing, the patient can grab the armrests on floor-based patient lifts or the walker. If using a ceiling-mounted patient lift, patient can grab parallel bars, if available. Release tension on the straps slightly to promote comfort and effective body movement.
9. If patient is steady, unlock brakes and instruct patient to walk as caregiver moves lift either by remote control or manually. (The patient can walk either facing the lift or facing away from the lift.)
10. When ambulation is completed, position the lift directly in front of bed or chair/wheelchair.
11. Lock brakes on floor-based patient lifts.
12. Instruct patient to back up until he or she feels bed or chair/wheelchair on the back of the legs, then to reach back for the bed or chair/wheelchair, and to lean forward to sit down. As patient sits, activate the motor to release the tension on the straps.
13. Detach the sling from the machine or instruct the patient to detach the straps. Remove the sling from the patient or instruct the patient to remove the sling. Avoid stooping to remove the sling. Never pull the sling roughly against the patient's skin.
14. Remove lifting device.

9.3

Ambulating
a patient at risk
for falls, using
a ceiling-mounted
patient lift

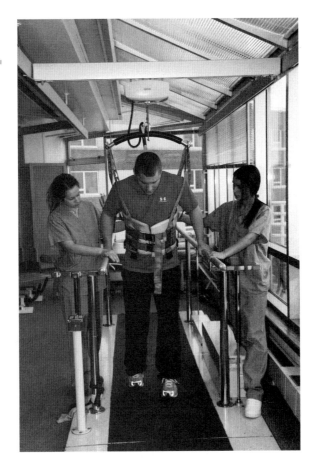

Bathing/Showering Out of Bed

Description of Task and Associated Risks

An individual with a chronic illness or physical disability may find it difficult to manage his or her own self-care. In the rehabilitation setting, self-care activities are referred to as activities of daily living, or ADLs. Some of the most common ADLs are eating, bathing, dressing, toileting, and grooming. The rehabilitation team will help individuals with chronic illnesses and physical disabilities develop skills needed to complete their ADLs as independently as possible. It may be necessary to use adaptive equipment to perform their ADLs. These are devices used to assist with completing activities that the individuals cannot perform as they did prior to their disability or illness. The amount of assistance needed to perform ADLs varies from person to person depending on motor impairment, sensory impairment, cognitive ability, and level of pain.

Bathing can include sponge bath, shower, or tub. These would also require the ability to wash upper or lower extremities and hair. Various pieces of adaptive equipment may be recommended to increase success and independence with bathing. Some examples include the following:

- Tub chair/tub bench with a back
- Bath and shower chair
- Grab bars
- Long-handled sponge
- Handheld shower
- Universal cuffs or other splints to assist with holding items
- Bath mitt with liquid soap or "soap on a rope"

Sitting balance and safety precautions should be addressed before attempting a shower on the shower chair. If balance is impaired, a reclining shower chair or a shower stretcher should be used. Risks to the caregiver include lifting heavy weights, awkward postures, long duration, reaching, and push/pull forces. Risks to the patient include skin shearing.

Patient Abilities

- One or more of the following:
  - ○ Physically unable to assist due to lack of weight-bearing ability
  - ○ Physically unable to assist due to lack of upper-extremity strength
  - ○ Unable to follow instructions
  - ○ Uncooperative

Resources Required

- One of the following:
  - ○ Ceiling-mounted lift with supine or seated hygiene sling
  - ○ Floor-based patient lift with seated hygiene sling (supine sling not available for this lift)
- Shower stretcher/trolley or commode/shower chair
- One or two caregivers (use two caregivers if the patient is uncooperative)
- Supplies for bathing

Technique 9-4

1. Follow *General Directions for All Tasks*.
2. Move shower stretcher/trolley or shower chair next to bed.
3. Select the appropriate hygiene sling for showering.
4. To attach sling to lift, lower head of bed flat if patient can tolerate.

Helpful Hint

Ideally, the equipment (shower stretcher/trolley and shower chair) should be adjusted to optimal height for the caregivers (elbow level), although not all brands include the height-adjustment function.

5. Apply sling using side-to-side rolling technique and right number of people; or, if patient is able to assist with upper extremities, instruct patient to assist with turning side to side. Place sling under patient. If sling is already in place, assess whether current sling position is appropriate for use.

6. Follow manufacturer's directions for applying the sling.

7. Attach sling to overhead attachment bar and activate motor to raise patient off the bed's surface.

8. Use manual or powered traverse to position patient over shower stretcher or shower chair, then lower the patient until contact is made.

9. Lower lift and remove sling straps. Leave the sling in position during shower.

10. Complete shower having patient participate to his or her maximum ability. To prevent reaching, wash patient's side of body closest to you and then move to the other side or turn shower stretcher or shower chair to complete the other side. A long-handled sponge could be used for the lower extremities in a shower chair to prevent bending and awkward posture.

11. Dry patient and cover with bath blanket when shower is completed.

12. Line the bed with one or two bath blankets.

13. Reattach straps to overhead attachment bar when shower is completed and activate motor to raise patient off shower stretcher or shower chair. Return patient to bed covered with bath blankets.

14. Lower lift and remove sling straps.

15. Dry back. Then remove sling and bath blanket using side-to-side rolling technique and right number of people; or, if patient is able to assist with upper extremities, instruct patient to assist with turning side to side.

16. Remove lift.

Special Transfer Approach for a Patient with a Lower Limb Amputation

Description of Task and Associated Risks

Patients with an amputation become structurally asymmetrical because there is an altered sensation and a loss of musculature on the amputated side (Tokuno, Sanderson, Inglis, & Chua, 2003. Together, these changes present challenges in mobility and daily activities. The center of gravity is shifted, significantly affecting balance. Ceiling lifts and floor-based lifts with the proper amputee sling can assist with transfers, sitting balance, trunk control, and strengthening the non-affected lower extremity. An amputee sling supports the whole body up to shoulder height and the pelvis region and is suitable

VIEW VIDEO 9.3: Transfer a Patient with a Lower Limb Amputation

for lifting both single and double above-the-knee amputees. It is important to select the right size. Risks to the caregiver include lifting heavy weights, awkward postures, reaching, and push/pull forces. Risks to the patient include skin shearing.

Patient Abilities

- Cannot bear weight on one or both legs
- Uncooperative or unable to follow instructions

Resources Required

- Floor-based patient lift or ceiling-mounted patient lift
- Amputee sling (amputation sling would be used for lifting both single and double above-knee amputations, as shown in picture)
- Wheelchair or chair
- Two caregivers

Technique 9-5

1. Follow *General Directions for All Tasks*.
2. Position and lock wheelchair next to bed.
3. Apply amputee sling using side-to-side rolling technique and right number of people; or, if patient is able to assist with upper extremities, instruct patient to assist. Place small repositioning sling under patient's back. If sling is already in place, assess whether current sling position is appropriate for use.
4. Follow manufacturer's directions for applying the sling.
5. Attach sling to overhead attachment bar, or instruct patient to attach straps to increase fine motor skills and finger, wrist, and upper-arm strength. Activate motor to raise patient off the bed's surface.
6. Encourage the patient to maintain proper body position to increase truck control.
7. Using manual or powered traverse to position patient over wheelchair, lower the patient until contact is made.
8. Lower lift and remove sling straps or instruct patient to remove straps.
9. Decide whether to remove the sling or leave it under the patient, considering the patient's skin integrity, tolerance of the sling surface, and length of time in the chair. If the patient is remaining in the chair for an extended period of time or has been transferred to the bed, then remove the transfer sling.
10. Do not leave the device hanging over the patient.

Case Study 9-1

The caregiver is caring for Mr. S, a 34-year-old male who was admitted to an acute care rehabilitation unit 1 week ago with a C6 spinal cord injury. Because of the level of injury, a bowel program was initiated. The patient's height is 5' 6" and weight is 160 lbs. The physician has ordered a suppository for every other morning. The patient's routine is up out of bed for meals and therapy in a reclining wheelchair. The patient has orthostatic hypotension and uses an abdominal binder and elastic stockings when out of bed.

Discussion Questions:

1. What safe patient-handling and movement equipment is appropriate for completing this patient's bowel program?
2. If that particular equipment is not available, what is the best action for you to take?
3. Before beginning the task, what steps would you take to complete the bowel program?
4. What patient handling and movement is involved with this task?

Post-Test Questions

9-1. Which of the following rehabilitation tasks involves heavy lifting and awkward posture?
   a. Neurogenic bowel care for an individual with a complete C4 spinal cord injury (SCI)
   b. Transferring an individual with multiple sclerosis (MS) with lower-extremity spasticity into a shower chair
   c. Putting compression stockings on an individual with a left cerebral vascular accident (CVA)
   d. All of the above

9-2. When a caregiver performs neurogenic bowel care for a patient in bed, what factors *most* contribute to risk?
   a. Holding the body in a side-lying position to access the rectum
   b. Twisting and reaching
   c. Pulling and pushing
   d. All of the above

9-3. What are the benefits of using safe patient-handling equipment in rehabilitation?
   a. Reduce the risk of musculoskeletal injuries in the caregiver.
   b. Reduce the risk of patient falls when ambulating patients.
   c. Equipment can be selected to match patient's functional ability as the patient progresses in the rehabilitation program.
   d. All of the above.

9-4. Which type of sling is the most appropriate for a tub bath for an individual with a T5 SCI?
   a. A supine sling is most appropriate.
   b. A hygienic seated sling is most appropriate for bathing.
   c. An ambulation sling is most appropriate.
   d. It is not safe for persons with an SCI to have a tub bath.

9-5. The primary function of a special amputee sling is to:
   a. Ambulate an individual with an above-the-knee amputation in preparation for a prosthesis
   b. Support the whole body up to shoulder height and pelvis region to prevent possible slip or fall due to shift in center of gravity and imbalance
   c. Reposition an individual with a below-the-knee amputation to a prone position to allow extension of the hip and knee of the residual leg
   d. None of the above

References

American Association of Spinal Cord Injury Nurses. (2007). *SCI: Neurogenic bowel care: Nursing guidelines*. Retrieved on January 4, 2008 from http://www.aascin.org/sci-neurogenic-bowel-care-nursing-guidelines.html.

Evitt, C. P., & Quigley, P. A. (2004). Fear of falling in older adults: A guide to its prevalence, risk factors and consequences. *Rehabilitation Nursing, 29*(6), 207–210.

Friedman, S. M., Munoz, B., West, S. K, Rubin, G. S., & Fried, L.P. (2002). Falls and fear of falling: Which comes first? A longitudinal prediction model suggests strategies for primary and secondary prevention. *Journal of American Geriatrics Association, 50*, 1329–1335.

Nelson, A., Tracey, C., Baxter, M., Nathenson, P., Rosario, M., Rockefeller, K., Joffe, M., Harwood, K. J., Whipple, K., & Le, H. (2005). Strategies to improve patient and healthcare provider safety in patient handling and movement tasks. *Rehabilitation Nursing, 30*(3), 80–83.

Tokuno, C. D., Sanderson, D. J., Inglis, T. J., & Chua, R. (2003). Postural and movement adaptations by individuals with a unilateral below-knee amputation during gait initiation. *Gait & Posture. 18* (3), 158–169.

Additional Reading

Derstine, J. B., & Drayton-Hargrove, S. (2001). *Comprehensive rehabilitation nursing*. Philadelphia: W. B. Saunders.

Consortium of Spinal Cord Medicine. (1998). Neurogenic bowel management in adults with spinal cord injury. Washington, DC: Paralyzed Veterans of America. Retrieved January 6, 2008 from http://www.pva.org.

Hoeman, S. P. (2002). *Rehabilitation nursing: Process, application, & outcomes* (3rd ed.). St. Louis, MO: Mosby.

Mauk, K. L. (2006). *Gerontological nursing: Competencies for care*. Sudbury, MA: Jones and Bartlett.

Mauk, K. L. (2007). *The speciality practice of rehabilitation nursing: A core curriculum* (5th ed.). Glenview, IL: Association of Rehabilitation Nurses.

Nelson, A. L. (Ed.). (2006). *Safe patient handling and movement: A practical guide for health care professionals*. New York: Springer.

Nelson, A., Harwood, K. J., Tracey, C. A., & Dunn, K. L. (2008). Myths and facts about safe patient handling in rehabilitation. *Rehabilitation Nursing, 33*(1), 10–17.

Rockefeller, K. (2008). Using technology to promote safe patient handling and rehabilitation. *Rehabilitation Nursing, 33*(1), 3–9.

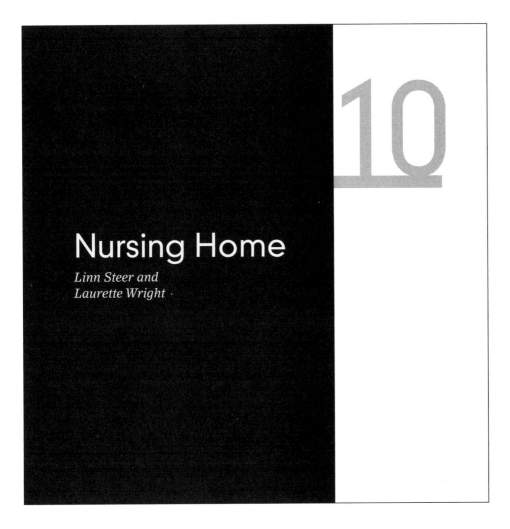

10

Nursing Home

Linn Steer and
Laurette Wright

Description of Setting

The nursing home may be residents' last home in life, so it is important that they feel at home and receive care that promotes dignity. At the same time, the nursing home is a workplace for the caregivers, who require safe working environments. This combination can be challenging, making it important to find solutions in the everyday care that works well for both parties. Note that the term *resident* will be used in this chapter rather than *patient* in order to emphasize that we are referring to people living in the facility.

Unique Challenges to Providing Safe Resident Handling in this Setting

Maintaining a person's mobility is crucial for maintaining dignity and quality of life. Immobility contributes to several adverse conditions, including deconditioning/muscle atrophy, dizziness, osteoporosis, constipation, incontinence, pressure ulcers, deep vein thrombosis (DVT), pulmonary embolism (PE), pneumonia, confusion, and depression (Weaver, 2005; Steer, 2005). In addition to improving outcomes, mobilizing residents has a positive effect on caregiver workload. Improving resident function contributes to independence, thereby eliminating many high-risk resident-handling tasks.

High-Risk Tasks

Specifically, high-risk tasks to be described include:

- Feeding a resident in bed
- Feeding a resident in a seated position
- Performing hygiene care in a seated position
- Transfer in/out of a geriatric dependency chair
- Repositioning in a geriatric dependency chair

Objectives

1. Describe the unique challenges associated with safe resident handling in nursing home settings.
2. Identify high-risk resident-handling tasks in nursing home settings.
3. For each high-risk resident-handling task, delineate the number of caregivers, types of equipment, and tips for performing the task safely.

Pre-Test Questions

10-1. Which of the following is *not* considered a high-risk task for a nursing home?
   a. Feeding a resident in bed or in a chair
   b. Performing hygiene care in a seated position
   c. Repositioning and transferring in/out of a dependency chair
   d. Placing patient in a standing shower

10-2. What resources are required to safely feed a nursing home resident in bed?
   a. A fixed-height bed
   b. A side table or over-bed table
   c. A height-adjustable working stool
   d. Both *b* and *c*

10-3. Which statement is true for dependency chairs?
   a. A dependency chair has three positions: seated, standing, and reclined.
   b. A dependency chair is always height-adjustable with removable armrests for ease in transfer.
   c. A dependency chair can be used instead of a wheelchair for mobility.
   d. A dependency chair should be used only for short periods of time.

10-4. Caregivers working in nursing homes spend approximately what percentage of their time assisting residents with feeding or administering medications?

a. 1% to 2%
b. 2% to 4%
c. 5% to 6%
d. 8% to 9%

10-5. While the caregiver is feeding nursing home residents, which of the following activities place the caregiver at risk for musculoskeletal injury?

a. Sustained awkward positions
b. Excessive reaching
c. Excessive bending
d. All of the above

10-6. The multipurpose hygiene chair can be used in many different ways. Which of the following purposes is *not* included in the use of a multipurpose hygiene chair?

a. A resting chair for dependent residents who need to use the bathroom facilities frequently
b. Toileting chair
c. Showering chair
d. Sleeping chair

General Directions for All Tasks

1. Complete *Assessment Criteria and Care Plan* for resident. Key assessment factors include physical ability to assist, ability to follow instructions, and cooperation. *Note: Weight and height may trigger use of bariatric algorithms.*
2. Review the algorithm for the high-risk resident-handling task to be performed and determine the number of caregivers, types of equipment, and techniques for performing each high-risk resident-handling task safely. If no algorithm exists, use the techniques described in this book to guide practice.
3. Check the weight capacity of the equipment to be sure it is able to handle the resident's weight.
4. Remove obstacles to performing the resident-handling tasks. Obstacles include too little room to maneuver the equipment, equipment stored on the floor posing a stumbling hazard, or inability to perform the activity without threats to resident dignity (e.g., lack of privacy). You may need to remove chairs or bed tables, separate beds, move floor-based equipment, and ask visitors to leave.
5. Make sure selected equipment is in good working order. If the equipment is battery operated, check that the battery is charged. Verify that the appropriate slings and attachments are available. Review safe operation of the equipment, including location of emergency buttons or manual controls for the event of a power failure.
6. Ensure sufficient caregivers are available to help, as specified in the algorithm.

7. Make sure beds are adjusted to caregiver's waist/elbow height before performing bed-related resident-handling tasks.
8. Explain the procedure to the resident and assisting caregivers.
9. Wear gloves according to proper infection-control practices and facility policies.

Feeding a Resident in Bed

Description of Task and Associated Risks

Caregivers spend approximately 5% to 6% of their time assisting with eating or drinking (Brinkhof & Knibbe, 2003). These activities can involve sustained awkward positions, as well as excessive reaching, bending, and twisting. Use of a height-adjustable bed or chair for the residents, combined with a height-adjustable working stool for the caregivers, can significantly reduce caregiver risk by increasing the time spent in a healthy position from 50% to at least 73% (Ibid).

In nursing home settings, it is also important to help the residents use their remaining abilities and promote mobility. If possible, the residents should get out of bed and sit together in the dining room. Fostering resident independence is key, even when the resident may perform slowly or when it requires effort to get the resident out of bed and to a common dining area.

Resident Abilities

- No upper-extremity strength and/or cognitively unable to follow instructions

Resources Required

- A height-adjustable working stool (The height-adjustable working stool should have casters and be easy to move around while someone is seated on it. It should be easy to raise and lower. The seat should preferably be of a saddle type to encourage a healthy back posture while making it possible to keep the feet on the ground even when in higher positions.)
- A side table or over-bed table
- Supplies for feeding: There are numerous eating and drinking devices that can be used to simplify both independent and assisted eating and drinking. Specially designed cutlery, plates, bowls, cups, and glasses are available to suit residents with various disabilities and can make the feeding activity much easier for both residents and staff.
- One caregiver

Technique 10-1

1. Follow *General Directions for All Tasks*.
2. Make sure the resident is positioned high enough to the head end of the bed to be able to sit up partially and also close enough to the side of the bed to avoid excessive reaching by the caregiver. Repositioning in bed is further

described in chapter 2. After making sure the resident's upper body is in a good position, use the bed function to raise the foot end (this function will prevent the resident from sliding down—see further details in the medical/ surgical chapter) and then the head end of the bed to an appropriate height (determined by the resident's condition and abilities).

3. Lower the bed to its lowest position.
4. Make sure the side table or over-bed table is put in a position that eliminates twisting of the upper body to collect the food and drinks. An over-bed table is preferable because it is then possible to place the food in front of the resident.

Helpful Hint

If you are right-handed, the resident should be close to you when you are sitting on the right side of the resident (from resident's perspective) and vice versa (see figure 10.2).

5. Place the food and drinks on the table.
6. Protect the bed linens and resident from any accidental spilling by placing a towel or similar covering on the resident.
7. Place the height-adjustable working stool close to the bed and sit down facing the resident. Adjust the height of the stool so your feet are placed firmly on the ground and you are in a good position to reach the resident without having to stand up. If necessary, use the wheels of the stool instead of leaning or twisting in order to collect the food or drinks.
8. Start feeding. Note that some residents eat very slowly. Let them take their time. Make sure you put down the spoon, glass, or equivalent to rest your shoulder in between each bite or sip.

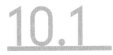

A height-adjustable working stool

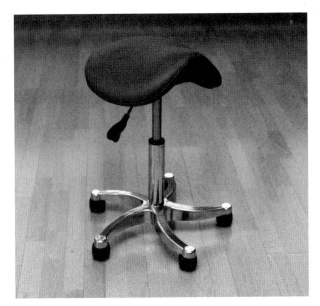

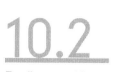

Feeding a resident
in bed

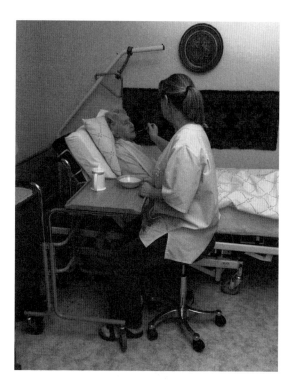

Feeding a Resident in a Seated Position

Description of Task and Associated Risks

Feeding a resident in a seated position can involve sustained awkward positions as well as excessive reaching, bending, and twisting. Use of a height-adjustable chair for the resident, combined with a height-adjustable working stool for the caregiver, can significantly reduce caregiver risk.

Resident Abilities

- Not cooperative or lacks upper-extremity strength

Resources Required

- A height-adjustable working stool
- One caregiver
- Supplies for feeding

Technique 10-2

1. Follow *General Directions for All Tasks*.
2. Make sure the resident is positioned appropriately in the chair or wheelchair (i.e., body follows the contours of the chair) and is sitting comfortably. Reposition the resident if necessary, as described in chapter 2.

3. Place the wheelchair on one side of a table corner with the resident facing the table and lock the breaks. If you are right-handed, the resident should be placed on your left side, and vice versa.

Helpful Hint

If you are right-handed, the resident should be placed on your left side, and vice versa.

4. Protect the resident's clothes by using a bib, napkin, towel, or similar.
5. Place the food and drinks in front of the resident.

Helpful Hint

Place the height-adjustable working stool on the right side of the resident if you are right-handed; otherwise, place it on the left side

6. Place the height-adjustable working stool on the right side of the resident if you are right-handed (otherwise, place it on the left side) on the other side of the table corner and sit down facing the resident (see figure 10.3). Adjust the height of the stool so your feet are placed firmly on the ground. If necessary, for example, if the wheelchair is too big to get close to the table, use the wheels of the working stool instead of leaning or twisting in order to collect the food or drinks.
7. Start feeding. Note that some residents eat very slowly. Let them take their time. Make sure you put down the spoon, glass, or equivalent to rest your shoulder in between each bite or sip.

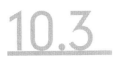

Feeding a resident in a wheelchair

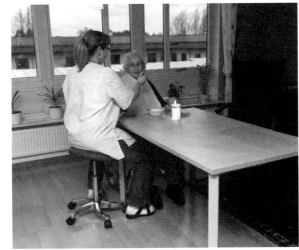

Performing Hygiene Care in a Seated Position

Description of Task and Associated Risks

Hygiene care in this case means all care tasks that can be included in the hygiene routines that take place in a nursing home (i.e., dressing, undressing, changing incontinence pads, washing certain body parts, full-body showering, hair washing, foot care, and toileting). Studies have shown that caregivers spend about 25% of the total nursing time on these activities during a normal shift (Brinkhof & Knibbe, 2003). Considering the excessive forces placed on the spine, neck, and shoulders during this task, it is important to make the right decisions on what hygiene equipment to use. Research shows that caregivers using a fixed-height hygiene chair for washing and showering residents work over 69% of the time in a potentially unhealthy posture (Knibbe & Knibbe, 1996). When washing, bathing, and showering residents on a height-adjustable bed (which is an excessively passive solution for residents who have the ability to sit up), caregivers spend about 61% of the time working in potentially harmful positions (Knibbe & Knibbe, 1994).

There are two types of seated height-adjustable hygiene solutions: multipurpose hygiene chairs and height-adjustable hygiene chairs.

Multipurpose hygiene chairs: As the name suggests, the multipurpose hygiene chair can be used for many different things. Apart from being a hygiene chair, it can also be used as a resting chair for dependent residents who need to go to the bathroom often. By placing accessory cushions in the chair, residents with, for example, feces incontinence can comfortably be taken to the toilet and partly showered off afterwards, without any additional transfers having to take place. The multipurpose hygiene chair can be placed over a toilet or used with a bedpan. A height-adjustable working stool can be a beneficial complement to the multipurpose hygiene chair, especially when working in the so-called care-raiser position.

View Video 10.1: Showering a Patient Using a Multi-Purpose Hygiene Chair

Helpful Hint

With a multipurpose hygiene chair, it is possible, via a hand control, to place the resident in three different positions: a normal seated position (Figure 10.4), a reclined position (Figure 10.5), or the care-raiser position (a position where the lower part of the resident's body is lifted—Figure 10.6), all at the preferred height. This last position makes it possible for one caregiver to dress and undress a resident safely and also change incontinence pads without having to use any other equipment.

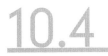

Hygiene care
performed with
patient in seated
position

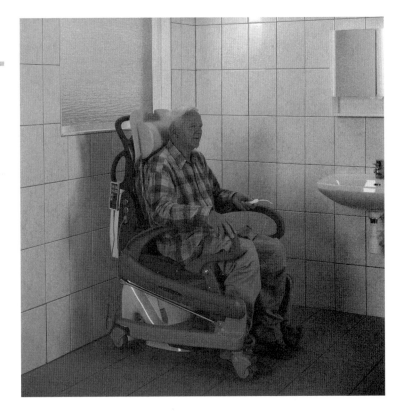

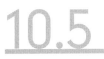

Hygiene care
performed with
patient in reclined
position

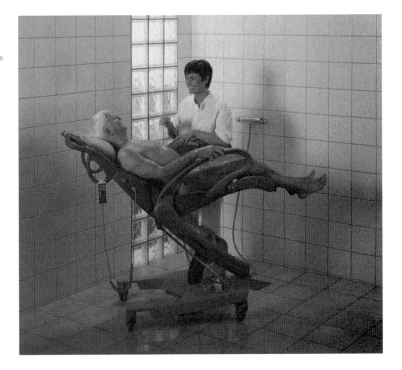

10.6

Hygiene care
performed with
patient in care-raiser
position

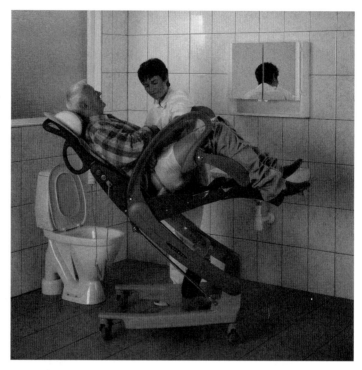

Height-adjustable hygiene chairs: There are many different height-adjustable hygiene chairs, both manual and powered. The common feature of all of them is that they can be adjusted in height. A height-adjustable hygiene chair should also have leg rests that allow for the feet to come up in an ergonomic position (see Figure 10.7). When in the highest position, the chair should either automatically be tilted back a little or should have a separate reclining function. This will both give better body access for the caregiver and a safer and more relaxing position for the resident.

View Video 10.2: Showering
a Patient Using a Height-
Adjustable Hygiene Chair

The main difference between the multipurpose hygiene chair and the height-adjustable hygiene chair is that the multipurpose hygiene chair provides access to the lower part of the body and thereby the increases the caregiver's ability to dress, undress, and change incontinence pads. For the more able residents who can either enter the hygiene chair by themselves or with help from a caregiver and a sit-to-stand lift (see Figure 10.8), it is possible to access the lower part of the body in a standing position before the resident enters and exits the chair. If a resident is feces incontinent but otherwise able to use a height-adjustable hygiene chair, it is advisable to use a multipurpose hygiene chair instead. This way it is convenient, both for the resident and caregiver, to clean and rinse the lower part of the body because this can be done without taking off the trousers and without any additional equipment. Just like the multipurpose hygiene chair, the height-adjustable hygiene chair can be placed over a toilet (see Figure 10.9) or can be used with a bedpan. It can also be used in combination with a height-adjustable working stool.

10.7

Leg rests lifting the feet to the right height

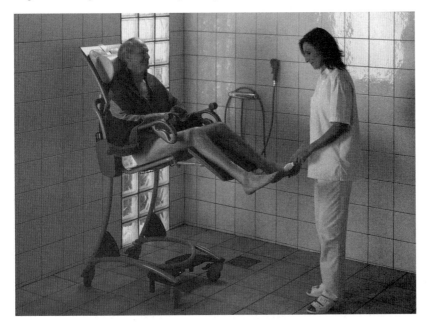

10.8

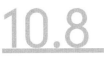

Assisting patient to hygiene chair using sit-to-stand lift

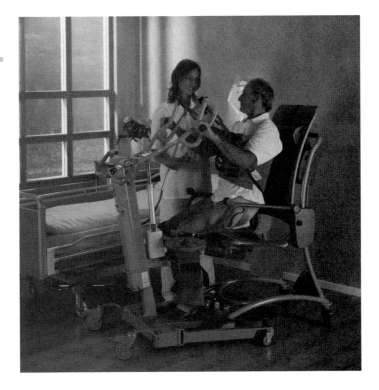

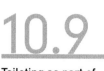

10.9

Toileting as part of
the hygiene routine

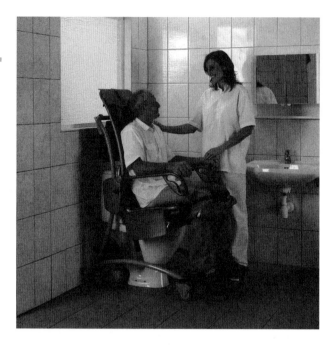

When using a height-adjustable hygiene chair with leg rests or a multipurpose hygiene chair, inexperienced users work in healthy positions for at least 75% of the time (59% without leg rests) (Brinkhof & Knibbe, 2003; Knibbe & Knibbe, 1994).

10.10

Percentage of time spent in a healthy working position when performing hygiene care using different nursing aids

Nursing aid	Percentage
Height-adjustable hygiene chair with legrests / Multi-purpose hygiene chair	74.8
Height-adjustable hygiene chair without legrests	58.8
Height-adjustable bath	56.3
Height-adjustable shower trolley	53.0
Fixed height bath	41.6
Height-adjustable bed	39.4
Fixed height shower trolley	38.6
Fixed height hygiene chair	31.4

When deciding how hygiene care, including undressing and dressing, should be performed with a resident, see Figure 10.11.

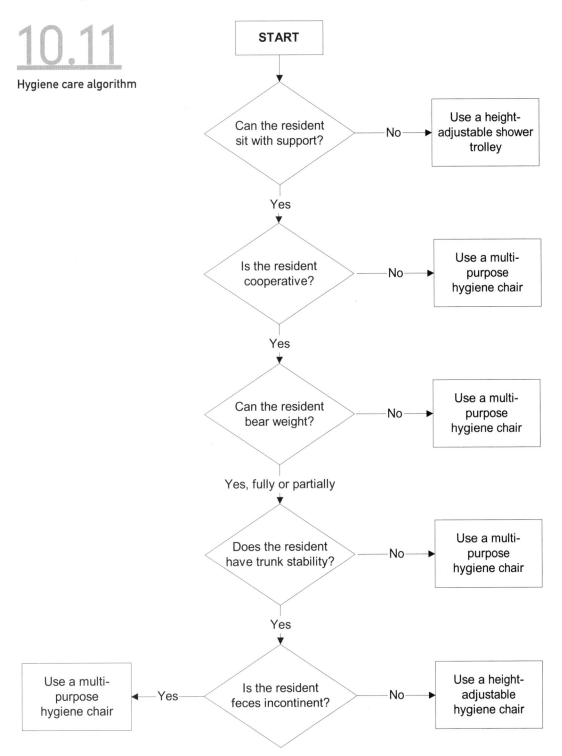

10.11

Hygiene care algorithm

Resident Abilities

- Can sit with support (symmetrical body position with 90 degrees flexion in hips and knees)
- (For further assessment, please see Appendix A, Algorithm 30.)

Resources Required

- A height-adjustable hygiene chair or multipurpose hygiene chair
- Resident-lifting device
  ○ A floor-based or ceiling-mounted resident lift
  ○ A powered sit-to-stand lift (if resident is able to use this)
- One–three caregivers (one caregiver can complete the task; additional caregivers might be needed if the resident is uncooperative or combative)

Technique 10-3

1. Follow *General Directions for All Tasks*.
2. Transfer the dressed resident into the hygiene chair using a suitable resident lift. When a resident is using a height-adjustable hygiene chair, the lower part of the body must be undressed before the resident sits down in the chair. Make sure the trousers and underwear are pulled down to at least knee level before the resident sits down. If incontinence pads are used, remove them as well. If the resident has the ability to stand but requires assistance to undress, it might be enough to hold on to a walking device, toilet armrests, or other handles situated in the hygiene area. If the resident requires a sit-to-stand lift, use Technique 2-4 (Appendix A, Algorithm 1) in chapter 2 (i.e., undress the lower part of the body before step 11). When using a multipurpose hygiene chair, the resident can be transferred fully dressed because complete undressing and dressing is possible in the chair. When using a sling lift, see the techniques in chapter 2 if you are transferring the resident from a bed to the multipurpose hygiene chair. If you are doing the transfer from a wheelchair, dependency chair, or similar, see technique below.
3. Ensure privacy by entering the hygiene area before the resident undresses.
4. Apply the wheel brakes once the resident is placed in the right position for showering or other hygiene-care activity.
5. Start with the chair in a sitting position at a comfortable height.
6. Remove the clothes on the upper body. A resident with trunk stability might be able to actively lean forward by holding on to the armrests and pulling himself/herself forward. If this is not possible, stand in front of the resident and pull him/her carefully toward you while removing the clothes.

When using a multipurpose hygiene chair:
7. Raise the chair, unbutton the trousers, and pull them down as far as possible. If the feet are in a high enough position, take off the shoes. Otherwise wait.
8. Bring the chair into the care-raiser position.

9. Pull down the trousers to the knees and if the resident uses incontinence pads, remove them by pulling them down from behind. This is also a good position from which to remove socks and compression stockings (see Technique 4-2 in chapter 4). Take off the shoes if this has not already been done.

10. Bring the chair back to a sitting position.

11. Take off the underwear and trousers.

12. The resident is now fully undressed and the showering procedure can begin. Start by bringing the chair once again into the care-raiser position.

13. Wash the lower parts of the body and rinse afterward.

14. Bring the chair back to a sitting position.

15. Get the resident to lean forward (see point 6 above), and wash the back.

16. Raise the chair and bring it into the fully reclined position. Wash and shower the rest of the resident's body in this position. Use a new cloth. Start with the hair and end with the feet. Make sure you adjust the height of the chair for a correct working posture during hair wash and pedicure. This is also a good position for shaving.

17. Dry the resident with a towel. Use a spare towel to cover the resident to prevent him/her from getting cold. Also make sure to dry the contact surfaces on the chair. Put on the incontinence pads, if used, and then put on the underwear, socks, compression stockings (see Technique 4-2 in chapter 4), and trousers. Pull up the underwear and trousers as far as possible.

18. Bring the chair to a (low) sitting position.

19. Dry the back of the resident and the chair's backrest.

20. Dress the upper part of the body (see point 6 above).

21. Raise the chair and bring it into the care-raiser position.

22. Dry the lower parts of the body and the chair seat. Complete putting on the incontinence pads, if used, and pull up the underwear and trousers. Put on the shoes.

23. Adjust the multipurpose hygiene chair back to a sitting position and lower the chair.

24. Release the brakes.

25. Ready for transportation and/or transfer out of the multipurpose hygiene chair.

When using a height-adjustable hygiene chair:

7. Raise the chair to a high position and remove the trousers, underwear, socks, compression stockings (see Technique 4-2 in chapter 4), and shoes. If leg rests are available, apply these to get the feet into a good, ergonomic position.

8. The resident is now fully undressed, and the showering procedure can begin.

9. Wash and shower the resident's body in this position. Start with the hair and end with the feet. Make sure you adjust the height of the chair for a correct working posture during hair wash and pedicure.

10. Dry the resident with a towel. Use a spare towel to cover the resident to prevent him/her from getting cold. Also make sure to dry the contact surfaces on the chair.

11. Put on the underwear, compression stockings (see Technique 4-2 in chapter 4), socks, trousers, and shoes. Pull up the underwear and trousers to knee height.

12. Take away the leg rests and bring the chair to a low position.

13. Wipe off the resident's back with a cloth and then dry it with a towel. Dry the chair's backrest.
14. Dress the upper part of the body (see point 6 above).
15. Get the resident to stand up using the same method as when entering the chair (see point 2 above). While the resident is in the standing position, dry the lower parts of the body. Put on the incontinence pads, if used, and pull up the underwear and trousers.
16. The resident is ready for transfer.

Helpful Hint

Make sure to inform the resident when you are changing position and what you are going to do next so he/she is prepared. Also promote mobility by making sure the resident is using his/her remaining abilities, e.g., washing and drying the face and upper body.

Transfer in/out of Geriatric Dependency Chair Using Sit-to-Stand Lift

Description of Task and Associated Risks

Dependency chairs are often an ideal choice for use in long-term care settings, particularly for allowing residents with moderate to severe restricted mobility to sit comfortably for prolonged periods of time while fulfilling pressure-reduction needs. In addition, this type of chair is an effective means of eliminating bed-chair-bed transfers by functioning as a wheelchair and recliner. Transferring residents in and out of dependency chairs poses risks to caregivers of lifting heavy loads, awkward postures, and frequency, while residents are at risk of skin shearing.

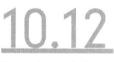

Dependency chair

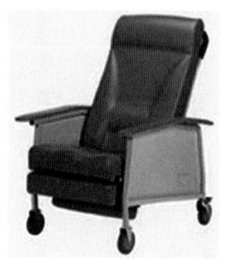

Resident Abilities

- Partially able to assist
- Cooperative
- Moderately stable in upper trunk
- Able to bear weight on at least one lower extremity

Resources Required

- A dependency chair (available in a wide range of models and styles but typically including three positions—upright, deep recline, and elevated leg rest/footrest—an overlap tray, enclosed side panels, and four rolling casters for easy transport by caregiver)
- Sit-to-stand lift
- Correct sling size and style
- Small friction-reducing device (FRD)
- Two caregivers

Technique 10-4

1. Follow *General Directions for All Tasks*.
2. Refer to Chapter 2 regarding use of sit-to-stand lift to transfer from bed to chair (Technique 2.4).
3. The model of the dependency chair and the sit-to-stand lift's ability to maneuver around the base of the dependency chair may limit the caregiver's ability to lower the resident in a position so that the resident's buttocks are aligned toward the rear of the dependency chair seat. To help solve this problem, if encountered, the caregiver may proceed as follows:
   a. Ensure that the brakes are applied to the dependency chair.
   b. Prior to placing the resident in the sit-to-stand lift, place an FRD directly against the seat of the dependency chair and place a drawsheet or pad on top of it. A portion of the FRD should drape over the edge of the dependency chair's seat.
   c. Push the lift and position it close enough to the chair so that the back of the resident's legs are touching the edge of the chair and lower him/her onto the chair seat.
   d. Apply the brake to the lift.
   e. Ensure that the resident's legs and feet are supported by the lift's platform and knee support. This will help stabilize the resident's legs and prevent him/her from sliding forward and onto the floor.
   f. Remove the sling and detach any straps located at the resident's legs.
   g. One caregiver on each side of resident grasps the edge of the resident's drawsheet/pad and pulls the resident backward to position toward the rear of the seat.
   h. Remove the FRD.
   i. Release the lift brake and remove the lift.
   j. Recline the chair and/or raise knee position (if available) to prevent the resident from sliding toward the front edge of the chair.

Transfer in/out of Geriatric Dependency Chair Using Resident Lifting Device (Floor-Based or Ceiling-Mounted)

Description of Task and Associated Risks

Residents in dependency chairs must be returned to bed in accordance with resident comfort, ability to tolerate prolonged sitting, and good nursing practice to prevent pressure ulcers. This task puts the caregiver at risk of lifting heavy loads, awkward postures, and pushing/pulling.

Resident Abilities

- Unable to assist
- Unable to understand simple commands
- Unable to bear weight

Resources Needed

- A dependency chair
- Floor-based or ceiling-mounted sling lift
- Correct sling size (typically a split-leg model)
- Small FRD
- Two caregivers

Technique 10-5

1. Follow *General Directions for All Tasks*.
2. Position dependency chair in reclined position. Ensure brakes are applied on the chair.

3. Have two staff members on each side of resident.
4. Insert small FRD underneath resident's incontinence pad/drawsheet. Avoid direct contact with resident's skin to avoid possible skin tears.
5. Ensure that the FRD is positioned underneath the head and upper trunk.

6. Each caregiver takes the edge of the full-body sling and positions it underneath the FRD using a sliding motion, until the edge of the sling is located at the resident's coccyx (base of the spine).

7. Gently raise the resident's legs and insert sling leg strap so that it is placed at the inner thigh. Avoid rubbing the sling directly against resident's skin (friction).

8. Remove the FRD once the sling has been properly applied.

9. Open the legs (chassis) of the floor-based resident lift (if not using a ceiling-mounted lift) and roll toward the resident, positioning the lift at the side of the chair. One leg of the floor lift will be either in front of the chair (if you are trying to pick the resident up out of the chair) or in back of the chair (if you are trying to position the resident all the way to the back of the chair). The second leg of the floor lift will be directly under the chair. This arrangement allows better access to the resident versus approaching directly in front of the chair.

10. Position the floor-based resident lift so that the spreader bar is just above and centered over the resident.

11. Lower the spreader bar until the shoulder attachment points can be connected to the sling shoulder attachment. Tilt the spreader bar forward until the sling leg pieces can be connected. (*Note: You may need to lower the spreader bar.*) Connect the leg pieces under the thighs by lifting one leg at a time.

Always check that all the sling attachments are fully in position before and during the lifting cycle, and maintain tension as the resident's weight is gradually taken up.

Helpful Hint: Caution

Be careful not to lower the spreader bar onto the resident.

12. Lift the resident using the handset control and adjust the spreader bar to a comfortable reclined position for transfer.

13. Transfer resident to bed.

14. Move into the desired position above the bed, adjusting the sling position as necessary. Then lower using the handset control.

15. Detach the sling leg attachment, followed by the shoulder attachment, when the resident's body weight is fully supported by the bed.

16. Move the floor-based resident lift away from the resident and bed before removing the sling from underneath the resident.

Repositioning in a Geriatric Dependency Chair

Description of Task and Associated Risks

Due to gravity and the resident's inability to maintain a good seated posture, the caregiver must frequently reposition the resident in the dependency chair.

This task involves lifting heavy loads, awkward postures, and bending. The resident is at risk of skin shearing.

Resident Abilities

- Unable to assist

Resources Needed

- A dependency chair
- One or two FRDs, depending on size of resident
- Two caregivers (may need 3 if resident is uncooperative)

Technique 10-6

1. Follow *General Directions for All Tasks.*
2. Apply brakes to the dependency chair.
3. Position the dependency chair in a reclined position.
4. Choose **only one method here.** Then proceed to step 5.

   Method One: Insert the FRDs under the resident's drawsheet/incontinence pad. The FRDs should be underneath the resident's head, shoulders, and buttocks area.
   Method Two: Fold individual FRDs lengthwise. Caregiver "A" inserts folded sheet horizontally underneath the resident's drawsheet/incontinence pad. Caregiver "B" performs the same technique on the opposite side. The folded edges of the FRDs should touch each other.

5. If the resident's heels are unprotected, place an additional FRD underneath the heels to prevent direct rubbing against the surface of the chair or chair linen.
6. Caregivers grasp the outer edges of the drawsheet/absorbent pad and ***pull upward*** toward the top of the chair. Do not lift the drawsheet/pad off the dependency chair surface.
7. Once the resident is repositioned, remove the FRD. You may consider placing a pillow under the resident's knees to prevent him or her from sliding downward toward the bottom of the chair if the chair remains in a reclined position.

Case Study 10-1

Mr. A is a 72-year-old hemiplegic man. He has been living in the nursing home post-stroke and has right-sided weakness of the arm and leg. The left side is functional, and his trunk stability is intact. He is aphasic, making it difficult to understand him, although he is cognitively intact and understands what people around him are saying. Mr. A weighs 170 lbs. He has bladder and bowel incontinence. He likes to be independent and is easily frustrated when the caregivers are not responding to his needs quickly enough or when he cannot communicate due to his aphasia. Mr. A can often be seen sitting in his wheelchair, moving up and down the corridor independently using his left arm and leg to propel himself.

Discussion Questions:

1. Explain the optimal hygiene solution for Mr. A, including the number of caregivers and types of equipment needed.
2. What method should be used to transfer Mr. A in and out of the hygiene chair?
3. Describe step by step how the hygiene routine should be implemented.
4. Identify strategies you would use to make the procedure more dignified for Mr. A and safe for the caregivers.

Post-Test Questions

10-1. Which of the following is *not* considered a high-risk task for a nursing home?
   a. Feeding a resident in bed or in a chair
   b. Performing hygiene care in a seated position
   c. Repositioning and transferring in/out of a dependency chair
   d. Placing patient in a standing shower
10-2. What resources are required to safely feed a nursing home resident in bed?
   a. A fixed-height bed
   b. A side table or over-bed table
   c. A height-adjustable working stool
   d. Both *b* and *c*
10-3. Which statement is true for dependency chairs?
   a. A dependency chair has three positions: seated, standing, and reclined.
   b. A dependency chair is always height-adjustable with removable arm-rests for ease in transfer.
   c. A dependency chair can be used instead of a wheelchair for mobility.
   d. A dependency chair should be used only for short periods of time.
10-4. Caregivers working in nursing homes spend approximately what percentage of their time assisting residents with feeding or administering medications?
   a. 1% to 2%
   b. 2% to 4%
   c. 5% to 6%
   d. 8% to 9%
10-5. While the caregiver is feeding nursing home residents, which of the following activities place the caregiver at risk for musculoskeletal injury?
   a. Sustained awkward positions
   b. Excessive reaching
   c. Excessive bending
   d. All of the above

10-6. The multipurpose hygiene chair can be used in many different ways. Which of the following purposes is *not* included in the use of a multipurpose hygiene chair?

a. A resting chair for dependent residents who need to use the bathroom facilities frequently

b. Toileting chair

c. Showering chair

d. Sleeping chair

References

Brinkhof, A., & Knibbe, N. (May, 2003). The ErgoStat Program: Pilot study of an ergonomic intervention to reduce static loads for caregivers. *Professional Safety USA, May 2003.*

Knibbe, N. E., & Knibbe, J. J. (November, 1996). Postural load of nurses during bathing and showering of patients: Results of a laboratory study. *Professional Safety USA, November 1996.*

Steer, L. (Ed.). (2005). *Arjo guidebook for architects and planners: Elderly care facilities.* Eslov, Sweden: ARJO AB.

Weaver, D. (2005). Helping individuals to maintain mobility. *Nursing & Residential Care, 7,* 8.

Additional Reading

Bell, F., Dalgity, M. E., Fennell, M. J., & Aitken, R. C. (1979). Hospital ward patient-lifting tasks. *Ergonomics, 22*(11), 1257–1273.

Chaffin D. B., Andersson G. B. J., & Martin B. J. (1999). *Occupational biomechanics* (3rd ed.). New York: Wiley & Sons.

Engels, J. A., van der Gulden, J. W. J., Senden, T. F., Hertog, C. A. W. M., Kolk, J. J., & Brinkhorst, R. A. (1994). Physical workload and its assessment among the nursing staff in nursing homes. *JOM, (36),* 338–345.

Garg, A., & Owen, B. (1992). Reducing back stress in nursing personnel: An ergonomic intervention in a nursing home. *Ergonomics, 35*(11), 1353–1375.

Hui, L., Ng, G. Y. F., Yeung, S. S. M., & Hui-Chan, C. W. Y. (2001). Evaluation of physiological work demands and low back neuromuscular fatigue on nurses working in geriatric wards. *Applied Ergonomics, 32,* 479–483.

Knibbe, J. J., & Knibbe, N. E. (2006). Monitoring the effects of the ergonomic covenants for workers in Dutch Healthcare. Maastricht, Netherlands: LOCOmotion.

Nelson, A. L. (Ed.) (2005). *Handle with care: A practice guide for safe patient handling and movement.* New York: Springer.

Owen, B. D., Keene, K., Olson, S., & Garg, A. (1995). An ergonomic approach to reducing back stress while carrying out patient handling tasks with a hospitalized patient. In M. Hagberg, F. Hoffman, U. Stoessel, & G. Westlander, *Occupational health for health care workers.* Landsberg, Germany: ECOMED.

Owen, B. (1987). The need for application of ergonomic principles in nursing. In S. Asfour (Ed.), *Trends in Ergonomics/Human Factors IV* (pp. 831–838). Holland: Elsevier Science Publishers B.V.

Schibye, B., & Skotte, J. (2000). The mechanical loads on the low back during different patient handling tasks. Proceedings of the IEA2000/HFES 2000 Conference (5, 785–788). Santa Monica, CA: The Human Factors and Ergonomics Society.

Smedley, J., Egger, P., Cooper, C., & Coggon, D. (1995). Manual handling activities and risk of low back pain in nurses. *Occupational and Environmental Medicine, 52,* 160–165.

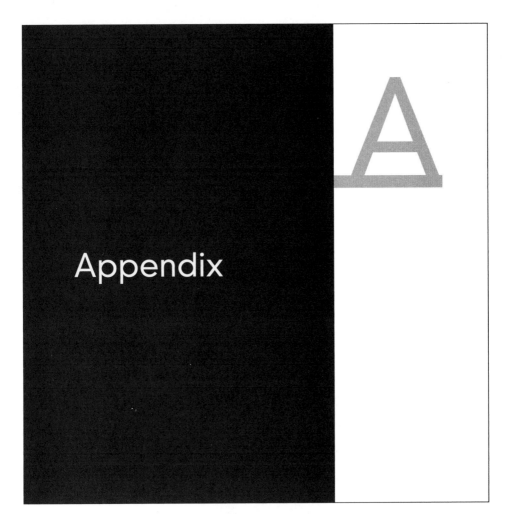

Appendix

Assessment Form _____

Standard Algorithms

Algorithm 1— Transfer to and From: Bed to Chair, Chair to Toilet, Chair to Chair, or Car to Chair _____

Algorithm 2— Lateral Transfer to and From: Bed to Stretcher, Trolley _____

Algorithm 3— Transfer to and From: Chair to Stretcher or Chair to Exam Table _____

Algorithm 4— Reposition in Bed: Side to Side, up in Bed _____

Algorithm 5— Reposition in Chair: Wheelchair and Dependency Chair _____

Algorithm 6— Transfer a Patient up From the Floor _____

Bariatric Algorithms

Algorithm 7— Bariatric Transfer to and From: Bed/Chair, Chair/Toilet, or Chair/ Chair _____

Algorithm 8— Bariatric Lateral Transfer to and From: Bed/ Stretcher/Trolley _____

Algorithm 9— Bariatric Reposition in Bed: Side to Side, up in Bed _____

Algorithm 10— Bariatric Reposition in Chair: Wheelchair, Chair or Dependency Chair _____

Algorithm 11— Bariatric Patient-Handling Tasks Requiring Access to Body Parts (Limb, Abdominal Mass, Gluteal Area) _____

Algorithm 12— Bariatric Transporting (Stretcher) _____

Algorithm 13— Toileting Tasks for the Bariatric Patient _____

Algorithm 14— Transfer a Bariatric Patient up From the Floor _____

Orthopaedic Algorithms

Algorithm 15— Turning Patient in Bed (Side to Side)—Patient with Orthopaedic Impairments _____

Algorithm 16— Vertical Transfer of a Postoperative Total Hip Replacement Patient (Bed to Chair, Chair to Toilet, Chair to Chair, or Car to Chair) _____

Algorithm 17— Vertical Transfer of a Patient With an Extremity Cast/Splint _____

Algorithm 18— Ambulation _____

Operating Room Algorithms

Algorithm 19— Lateral Transfer From Stretcher to and From the OR Bed _____

Algorithm 20— Positioning and Repositioning the Patient on the OR Bed to and From the Supine Position _____

Algorithm 21— Lifting and Holding Legs, Arm and Heads for Prepping in a Periop-erative Setting _____

Algorithm 22— Prolonged Standing _____

Algorithm 23— Retraction _____

Assessment Criteria and Care Plan for Safe Patient Handling and Movement

I. Patient's Level of Assistance:

_____ Independent— Patient performs task safely, with or without staff assistance, with or without assistive devices.

_____ Partial Assist—Patient requires no more help than standby, cueing, or coaxing, or caregiver is required to lift no more than 35 lbs of a patient's weight.

_____ Dependent—Patient requires nurse to lift more than 35 lbs of the patient's weight, or patient is unpredictable in the amount of assistance offered. In this case assistive devices should be used.

An assessment should be made prior to each task if the patient has varying level of ability to assist due to medical reasons, fatigue, medications, etc. When in doubt, assume the patient cannot assist with the transfer/repositioning.

II. Weight-Bearing Capability

_____ Full

_____ Partial

_____ None

III. Bilateral Upper-Extremity Strength

_____ Yes

_____ No

IV. Patient's level of cooperation and comprehension:

_____ Cooperative—may need prompting; able to follow simple commands.

_____ Unpredictable or varies (patient whose behavior changes frequently should be considered as unpredictable), not cooperative, or unable to follow simple commands.

V. Weight: _____ Height: _____

Body Mass Index (BMI) [needed if patient's weight is over 300 lbs][1]:_____

If BMI exceeds 50, institute Bariatric Algorithms

The presence of the following conditions are likely to affect the transfer/repositioning process and should be considered when identifying equipment and technique needed to move the patient.

VI. Check applicable conditions likely to affect transfer/repositioning techniques.

_____ Hip/Knee/Shoulder Replacements	_____ Respiratory/ Cardiac Compromise	_____ Fractures
_____ History of Falls	_____ Wounds Affecting Transfer/Positioning	_____ Splints/Traction
_____ Paralysis/Paresis	_____ Amputation	_____ Severe Osteoporosis
_____ Unstable Spine	_____ Urinary/Fecal Stoma	_____ Severe Pain/Discomfort
_____ Severe Edema	_____ Contractures/Spasms	_____ Postural Hypotension
_____ Very Fragile Skin	_____ Tubes (IV, Chest, etc.)	

Comments: _____

_____

_____

VII. Appropriate Lift/Transfer Devices Needed:

Vertical Lift: _____

_____

Horizontal Lift: _____

_____

Other Patient Handling Devices Needed: _____

_____

Sling Type: Seated_____ Seated (Amputee)_____ Standing_____ Supine_____ Ambulation_____
       Limb Support_____
Sling Size: _____
Signature: _____   **Date:** _____

[1]If patient's weight is over 300 lbs, the BMI is needed. For Online BMI table and calculator, see the National Heart Lung and Blood Institute Web site, nhlbi.nih.gov.

A.1

Algorithm 1: Transfer to and from: Bed to Chair, Chair to Toilet,
Chair to Chair, or Car to Chair

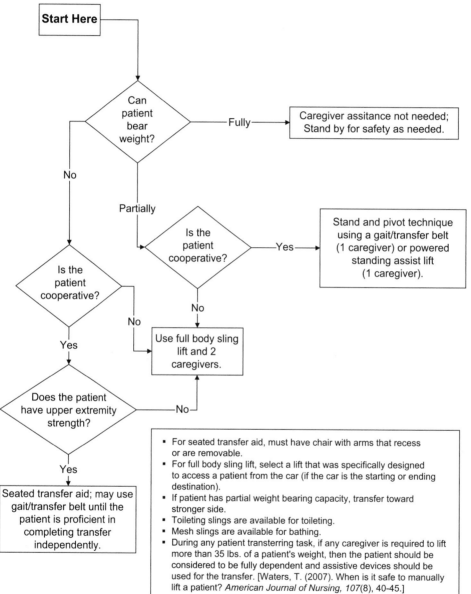

A.2

Algorithm 2: Lateral Transfer to and from: Bed to Stretcher, Trolley

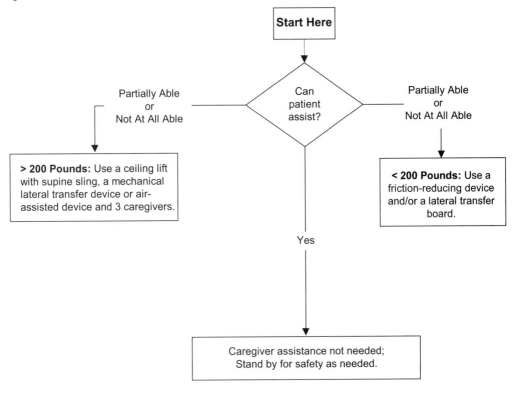

Start Here

Can patient assist?

Partially Able
or
Not At All Able

Partially Able
or
Not At All Able

> 200 Pounds: Use a ceiling lift with supine sling, a mechanical lateral transfer device or air-assisted device and 3 caregivers.

< 200 Pounds: Use a friction-reducing device and/or a lateral transfer board.

Yes

Caregiver assistance not needed;
Stand by for safety as needed.

- Destination surface should be 1/2" lower for all lateral patient moves.
- For patients with Stage III or IV pressure ulcers, care must be taken to avoid shearing force.
- During any patient transferring task, if any caregiver is required to lift more than 35 lbs of a patient's weight, then then patient should be considered to be fully dependent and assistive devices should be used for the transfer. (Waters, T. [2007]. When is it safe to manually lift a patient? *American Journal of Nursing, 107* [8], 53-59.)

A.3

Algorithm 3: Transfer to and from: Chair to Stretcher or Chair to Exam Table

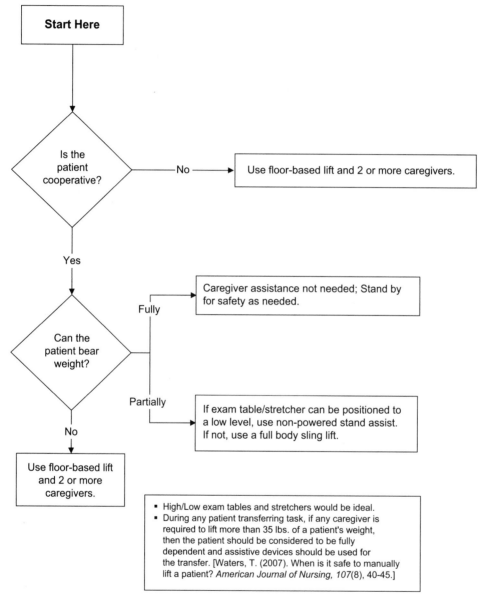

- High/Low exam tables and stretchers would be ideal.
- During any patient transferring task, if any caregiver is required to lift more than 35 lbs. of a patient's weight, then the patient should be considered to be fully dependent and assistive devices should be used for the transfer. [Waters, T. (2007). When is it safe to manually lift a patient? *American Journal of Nursing, 107*(8), 40-45.]

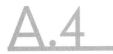

Algorithm 4: Reposition in Bed: Side to Side, up in Bed

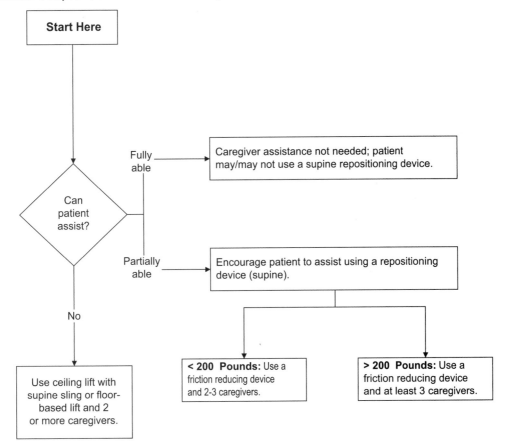

- This is not a one person task: DO NOT PULL FROM HEAD OF BED.
- When pulling a patient up in bed, the bed should be flat or in a Trendelenburg position (when tolerated) to aid in gravity, with the side rail down.
- For patients with Stage III or IV pressure ulcers, care should be taken to avoid shearing force.
- The height of the bed should be appropriate for staff safety (at the elbows).
- If the patient can assist when repositioning "up in bed," ask the patient to flex the knees and push on the count of three.
- During any patient handling task, if the caregiver is required to lift more than 35 lbs. of a patient's weight, then the patient should be considered to be fully dependent and assistive devices should be used.
  [Waters, T. (2007). When is it safe to manually lift a patient? *American Journal of Nursing, 107*(8), 40-45.]

A.5

Algorithm 5: Reposition in Chair: Wheelchair and Dependency Chair

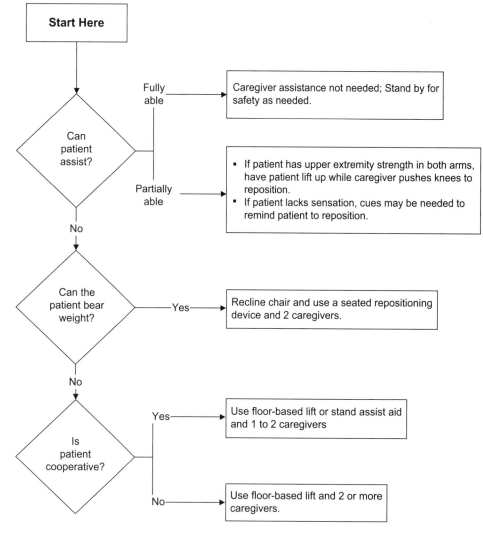

- Take full advantage of chair functions, e.g., chair that reclines, or use arm rest of chair to facilitate repositioning.
- Make sure the chair wheels are locked.
- During any patient transferring task, if any caregiver is required to lift more than 35 lbs. of a patient's weight, then the patient should be considered to be fully dependent and assistive devices should be used. [Waters, T. (2007). When is it safe to manually lift a patient? *American Journal of Nursing, 107*(8), 40-45.]

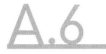

Algorithm 6: Transfer a Patient up from the Floor

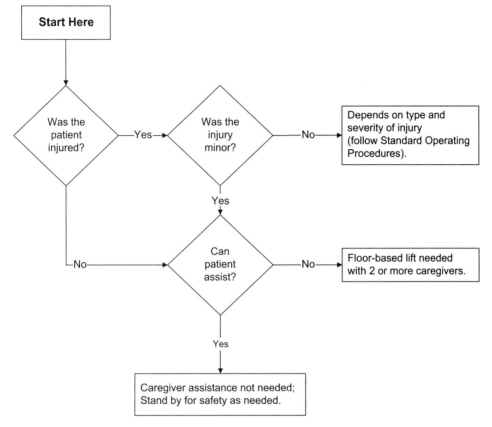

- Use floor-based lift that goes all the way down to the floor (most of the newer models are capable of this).
- During any patient transferring task, if any caregiver is required to lift more than 35 lbs. of a patient's weight then the patient should be considered to be fully dependent and assistive devices should be used. [Waters, T. (2007). When is it safe to manually lift a patient? *American Journal of Nursing, 107*(8), 40-45.]

A.7

Algorithm 7: Bariatric Transfer to and from: Bed/Chair, Chair/Toilet, or Chair/Chair

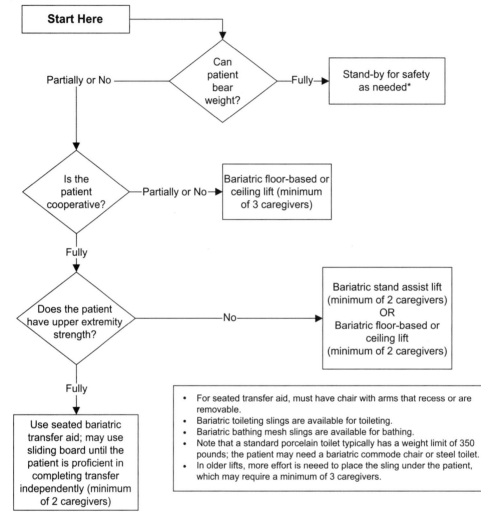

* "Stand-by for safety." In most cases, if a bariatric patient is about to fall, there is very little that the caregiver can do to prevent the fall. The caregiver should be prepared to move any items out of the way that could cause injury, try to protect the patient's head from striking any objects or the floor and seek assistance as needed once the person has fallen.
* If patient has partial weight-bearing capability, transfer toward stronger side.
* Consider using an abdominal binder if the patient's abdomen impairs a patient handling task.
* Assure equipment used meets weight requirements. Standard equipment is generally limited to 250-350 lbs. Facilities should apply a sticker to all bariatric equipment with "EC" (for expanded capacity) and a space for the manufacturer's rated weight capacity for that particular equipment model.
* Identify a leader when performing tasks with multiple caregivers. This will assure that the task is synchronized for increased safety of the healthcare provider and the patient.
* During any patient transferring task, if any caregiver is required to lift more than 35 lbs of a patient's weight, then the patient should be considered to be fully dependent and assistive devices should be used for the transfer.

A.8

Algorithm 8: Bariatric Lateral Transfer to and from: Bed/Stretcher/Trolley

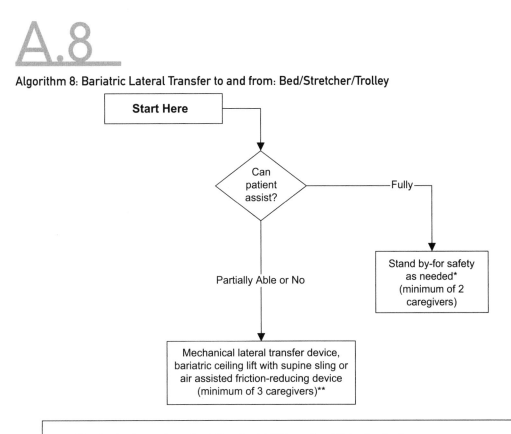

- The destination surface should be about 1/2" lower for all lateral patient moves.
- Avoid shearing force.
- Make sure bed is the right width, so excessive reaching by caregiver is not required.
- Lateral transfers should not be used with speciality beds that interfere with the transfer. In this case, use a bariatric ceiling lift with supine sling.
- Ensure bed or stretcher doesn't move with the weight of the patient transferring.
- ** Use a bariatric stretcher or trolley if patient exceeds weight capacity of traditional equipment.

---

* "Stand-by for safety." In most cases, if a bariatric patient is about to fall, there is very little that the caregiver can do to prevent the fall. The caregiver should be prepared to move any items out of the way that could cause injury, try to protect the patient's head from striking any objects or the floor and seek assistance as needed once the person has fallen.

* Assure equipment used meets weight requirements. Standard equipment is generally limited to 250-350 lbs. Facilities should apply a sticker to all bariatric equipment with "EC"(for expanded capacity) and a space for the manufacturer's rated weight capacity for that particular equipment model.

- If patient has partial weight-bearing capability, transfer toward stronger side.
- Consider using an abdominal binder if the patient's abdomen impairs a patient handling task.
- Identify a leader when performing tasks with multiple caregivers. This will assure that the task is synchronized for increased safety of the healthcare provider and the patient.
- During any patient transferring task, if any caregiver is required to lift more than 35 lbs of a patient's weight, then the patient should be considered to be fully dependent and assistive devices should be used for the transfer.

A.9

Algorithm 9: Bariatric Reposition in Bed: Side to Side, up in Bed

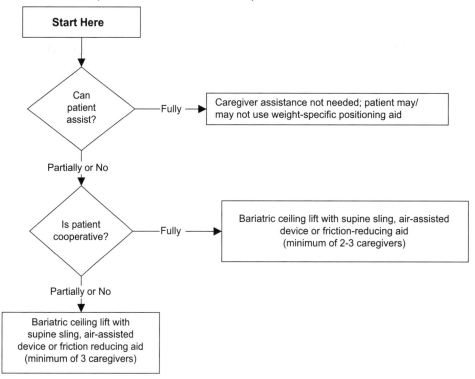

- When pulling a patient up in bed, place the bed flat or in a Trendelenburg position (if tolerated and not medically contraindicated) to aid in gravity; the side rail should be down.
- Avoid shearing force.
- Adjust the height of the bed to elbow height.
- Mobilize the patient as early as possible to avoid weakness resulting from bed rest. This will promote patient independence and reduce the number of high risk tasks caregivers will provide.
- Consider leaving a friction-reducing device covered with drawsheet, under patient at all times to minimize risk to staff during transfers as long as it doesn't negate the pressure relief qualities of the mattress/overlay.
- Use a sealed, high-density, foam wedge to firmly reposition patient on side. Skid-resistant texture materials vary and come in set shapes and cut-your-own rolls. Examples include:
    - Dycem (TM)
    - Scoot-Guard (TM): antimicrobial; clean with soap and water, air dry.
    - Posey-Grip (TM): Posey-Grip does not hold when wet. Washable, reusable, air dry.

- If patient has partial weight-bearing capability, transfer toward stronger side.
- Consider using an abdominal binder if the patient's abdomen impairs a patient handling task.
- Assure equipment used meets weight requirements. Standard equipment is generally limited to 250-350 lbs. Facilities should apply a sticker to all bariatric equipment with "EC" (for expanded capacity) and a space for the manufacturer's rated weight capacity for that particular equipment model.
- Identify a leader when performing tasks with multiple caregivers. This will assure that the task is synchronized for increased safety of the healthcare provider and the patient.
- During any patient handling task, if any caregiver is required to lift more than 35 lbs of a patient's weight, then the patient should be considered to be fully dependent and assistive devices should be used.

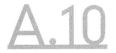
A.10

Algorithm 10: Bariatric Reposition in Chair: Wheelchair, Chair, or Dependency Chair

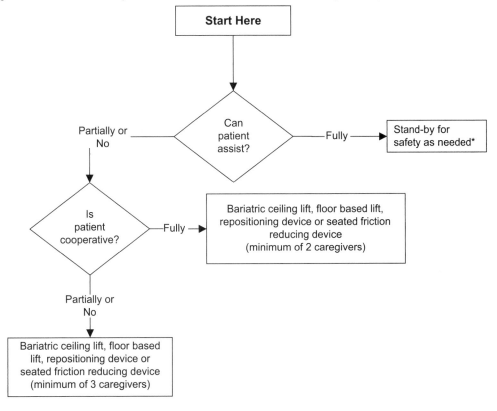

- Take full advantage of chair functions, e.g., chair that reclines, or use an arm rest of chair to facilitate repositioning.
- Make sure the chair wheels are locked.
- Consider leaving the sling under the patient at all times to minimize risk to staff during transfers after carefully considering skin risk to patient and the risk of removing/replacing the sling for subsequent moves.

- *   "Stand-by for safety." In most cases, if a bariatric patient is about to fall, there is very little that the caregiver can do to prevent the fall. The caregiver should be prepared to move any items out of the way that could cause injury, try to protect the patient's head from striking any objects or the floor and seek assistance as needed once the person has fallen.
- If patient has partial weight-bearing capability, transfer toward stronger side.
- Consider using an abdominal binder if the patient's abdomen impairs a patient handling task.
- Assure equipment used meets weight requirements. Standard equipment is generally limited to 250-350 lbs. Facilities should apply a sticker to all bariatric equipment with "EC" (for expanded capacity) and a space for the manufacturer's rated weight capacity for that particular equipment model.
- Identify a leader when performing tasks with multiple caregivers. This will assure that the task is synchronized for increased safety of the healthcare provider and the patient.
- During any patient transferring task, if any caregiver is required to lift more than 35 lbs of a patient's weight, then the patient should be considered to be fully dependent and assistive devices should be used for the transfer.

A.11

Algorithm 11: Bariatric Patient-Handling Tasks Requiring Access to Body Parts (Limb, Abdominal Mass, Gluteal Area)

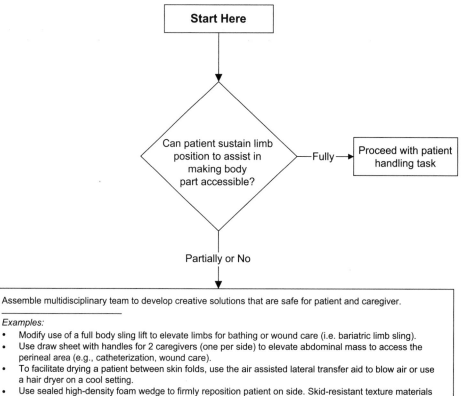

Start Here

Can patient sustain limb position to assist in making body part accessible? —Fully→ Proceed with patient handling task

Partially or No

Assemble multidisciplinary team to develop creative solutions that are safe for patient and caregiver.

Examples:
- Modify use of a full body sling lift to elevate limbs for bathing or wound care (i.e. bariatric limb sling).
- Use draw sheet with handles for 2 caregivers (one per side) to elevate abdominal mass to access the perineal area (e.g., catheterization, wound care).
- To facilitate drying a patient between skin folds, use the air assisted lateral transfer aid to blow air or use a hair dryer on a cool setting.
- Use sealed high-density foam wedge to firmly reposition patient on side. Skid-resistant texture materials vary and come in set shapes and cut-your-own rolls. Examples include:
  - Dycem(TM)
  - Scoot-Guard(TM): antimicrobial; clean with soap and water, air dry.
  - Posey-Grip(TM): Posey-Grip does not hold when wet. Washable, reusable, air dry.

- A multidisciplinary team needs to problem solve these tasks, communicate to all caregivers, refine as needed and perform consistently.
- Consider using an abdominal binder if the patient's abdomen impairs a patient handling task.
- During any patient transferring task, if any caregiver is required to lift more than 35 lbs of a patient's weight, then the patient should be considered to be fully dependent and assistive devices should be used for the transfer.

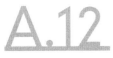

Algorithm 12: Bariatric Transporting (Stretcher)

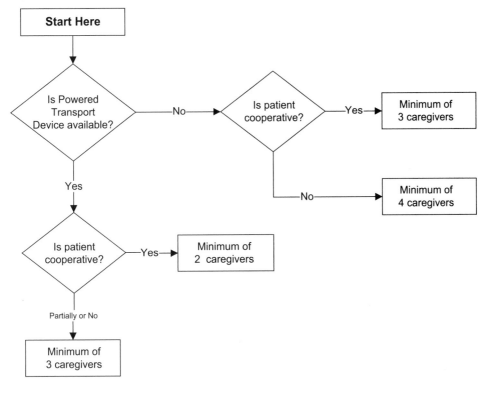

- If the patient has respiratory distress, the stretcher must have the capability of maintaining a high Fowler's position.
- Newer equipment often is easier to propel.
- If patient is uncooperative, secure patient in stretcher.
- During any patient transferring task, if any caregiver is required to lift more than 35 lbs of a patient's weight, then the patient should be considered to be fully dependent and assistive devices should be used for the transfer.

A.13

Algorithm 13: Toileting Tasks for the Bariatric Patient

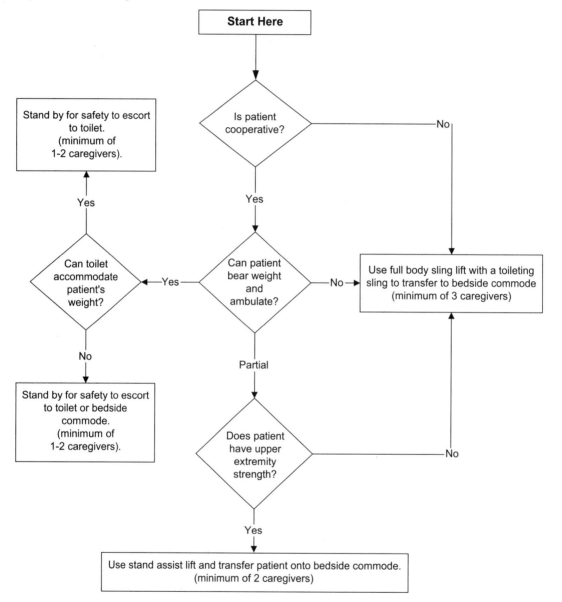

Considerations:
➤ Is bathroom doorway wide enough to accommote entry of mechanical lift device and patient?
➤ Assure equipment used meets weight requirements and is appropriately sized for patient.
➤ Typically, standard toilets are rated to 350 lbs. maximum capacity.
➤ During any patient transferring task, if any caregiver is required to lift more than 35 lbs. of a patient's weight, then the patient should be considered to be fully dependent and assistive devices should be used for the transfer.

A.14

Algorithm 14: Transfer a Bariatric Patient up from the Floor

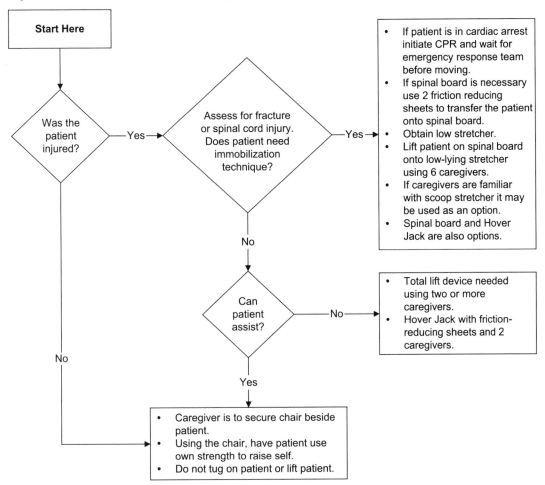

Start Here	• If patient is in cardiac arrest initiate CPR and wait for emergency response team before moving. • If spinal board is necessary use 2 friction reducing sheets to transfer the patient onto spinal board. • Obtain low stretcher. • Lift patient on spinal board onto low-lying stretcher using 6 caregivers. • If caregivers are familiar with scoop stretcher it may be used as an option. • Spinal board and Hover Jack are also options.

Was the patient injured? —Yes→ **Assess for fracture or spinal cord injury. Does patient need immobilization technique?** —Yes→

No ↓

Can patient assist? —No→
- Total lift device needed using two or more caregivers.
- Hover Jack with friction-reducing sheets and 2 caregivers.

No ↓ (from Was the patient injured?)

Yes ↓ (from Can patient assist?)

- Caregiver is to secure chair beside patient.
- Using the chair, have patient use own strength to raise self.
- Do not tug on patient or lift patient.

- Do **not** lift patient off floor.
- Do not allow patient to lean on caregiver for base of support.
- "Immobilization Technique" definition: use spinal precautions if can't use lift due to suspect hip, pelvic, or vertebral fractures.
- Use floor-based lift that goes all the way down to the floor (most of the newer models are capable of this).
- During any patient transferring task, if any caregiver is required to lift more than 35 lbs. of a patient's weight then the patient should be considered to be fully dependent and assistive devices should be used. [Waters, T. (2007). When is it safe to manually lift a patient? *American Journal of Nursing, 107*(8), 40-45.]

A.15

Algorithm 15: Turning Patient in Bed (Side to Side)—Patient with Orthopaedic Impairments

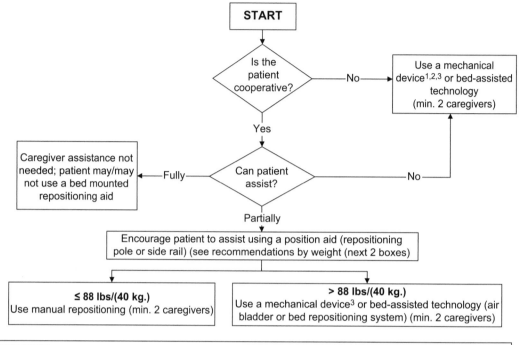

FOOTNOTES:
1. Maintain orthopaedic precautions as prescribed while performing this activity such as total hip, knee, shoulder, or spine precautions.
2. Select sling to meet and maintain the patient's pre-op or post-op positioning guideline/precautions for the affected limb/body part(s). For more information on sling section, see the "Slings Toolkit" at http://www.visn8.med.va.gov/patientsafetycenter/safePtHandling.
3. Examples of repositioning mechanical devices are: **Turning clips:** these simple slips attach to a bed sheet and can be used with a floor-based life or ceiling-based lift to facilitate turning a patient. **Turning straps/slings:** one end of these straps or slings is connected to the bed and the other end is attached to either a ceiling or floor based lift to facilitate turning the patient. **Powered mechanical devices:** a ceiling lift is a powered overhead lift that can be used with a repositioning sling to turn a patient in bed. **Friction reducing devices:** either tubular in design, or two separate pieces of material are placed under the patient to assist in turning the patient in bed or moving the patient to the head of the bed. **Pulley systems:** these devices work by use of a pulley system and an overhead frame. The user turns a crank, which engages the pulley system to retract straps that are connected to a rod and bed sheet, thus turning the patient on the side.

GENERAL NOTES:
- For any patient who has, or is at risk for a pressure ulcer, care should be taken to avoid shearing force (such as using a friction reducing device for repositioning in bed). Shearing force is when there are two forces moving in opposite directions adjacent to each other (like scissors).
- The height of the bed should be appropriate for staff safety (at elbow height).
- During any patient handling task, if the caregiver is required to lift more than 35 lbs./(16 kg.) of a patient's weight, then the patient should be considered fully dependent and an assistive device should be used. (Waters, T. [2007]. When is it safe to manually lift a patient? *American Journal of Nursing, 107*(8), 40-45.)

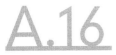

Algorithm 16: Vertical Transfer of a Postoperative Total Hip Replacement Patient (Bed to Chair, Chair to Toilet, Chair to Chair, or Car to Chair)

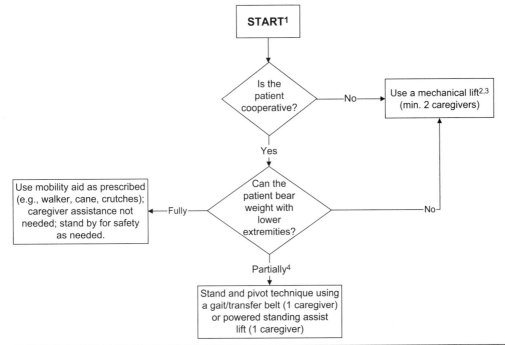

FOOTNOTES:

1. See 1A, 1B, 1C, 1D below for techniques to position patient at side of bed.

   1A. Moving from supine head of bed elevated to sitting at edge of bed requires: Patient's ability to shift their seated weight in a sitting position. Typically accomplished by unweighting one buttock and moving it toward the edge of the bed; repeating this in alternating fashion until patient is sitting at edge of bed.

   1B. With an impaired upper or lower extremity, caregiver might need to support the limb while patient attempts #1A.

   1C. If patient is unable to accomplish #1A with #1B and the amount of assistance from caregiver will exceed 35 lbs., then a mechanlical lift device should be used to achive sitting position at the edge of the bed.

   1D. Anti friction sheets and seated discs might be useful when the amount of caregiver assistanace is close to recommended limits; be aware of skin shearing risks. Shearing forces are caused when there are two forces moving in opposite directions adjacent to each other (like scissors).

2. Maintain orthopaedic precautions as prescribed while performing this activity such as total hip, knee, shoulder, or spine precautions.

3. Select sling to meet and maintain the patient's pre-op or post-op positioning guideline/precautions for the affected limb/body part(s). For more information on sling section, see the "Slings Toolkit" at http://www.visn8.med.va.gov/patientsafetycenter/safePtHandling.

4. This will include situations where the patient may be allowed:

   a) Limited weight bearing on one lower extremity and full weight bearing on the other extremity;

   b) Partial weight bearing through both lower extremities.

GENERAL NOTES:

- If patient has partial weight bearing capacity, transfer toward stronger side.
- For car transfers: a) If patient cannot tolerate a seated position when doing a car transfer use a stretcher transfer or alternative transportation may be required; b) All car transports should comply with state laws for both children and adults; c) Don't forget to use all of the features of the car (ie., adjustability of the seat) during the transfer.
- The height of the bed should be appropriate for staff safety (at elbow height).
- During any patient handling task, if the caregiver is required to lift more than 35 lbs./(16 kg.) of a patient's weight, then the patient should be considered fully dependent and an assistive device should be used.
  (Waters, T. [2007]. When is it safe to manually lift a patient? *American Journal of Nursing*, 107(8), 40-45.)

A.17

Algorithm 17: Vertical Transfer of a Patient with an Extremity Cast/Splint

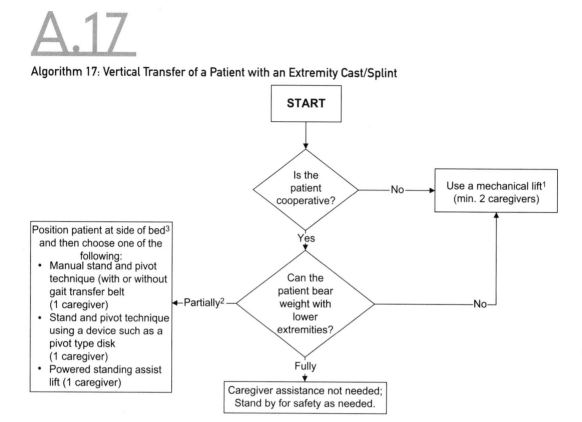

FOOTNOTES:
1. Select sling to meet and maintain the patient's pre-op or post-op positioning guideline/precautions for the affected limb/body part(s). For more information on sling section, see the "Slings Toolkit" at http://www.visn8.med.va.gov/patientsafetycenter/safePtHandling.
2. This will include situations where the patient may be allowed: a) Limited weight bearing on one lower extremity and full weight bearing on the other extremity; b) Partial weight bearing through both lower extremities.
3. (See 3A, 3B, 3C, 3D below)
3A. Moving from supine HOB elevated to sitting at edge of bed requires: Patient's ability to shift their seated weight in a sitting position. Typically accomplished by unweighting one buttock and moving it toward the edge of the bed repeating this in alternating fashion, until patient is sitting at edge of bed.
3B. With an impaired upper or lower extremity, caregiver might need to support the limb while patient attempts #1A.
3C. If patient is unable to accomplish #1A with #1B and the amount of assistance from caregiver will exceed 35 lbs., then a mechanical lift device should be used to achive sitting position at the edge of the bed.
3D. Anti friction sheets and seated discs might be useful; be aware of skin shearing risks. Shearing is caused when there are two forces moving in opposite directions adjacent to each other (like scissors).

GENERAL NOTES
- Need to test the fit of the sling with an immobilized arm.
- Maintain affected upper extremity immobilization/alignment.
- During any patient handling task, if the caregiver is required to lift more than 35 lbs./(16 kg.) of a patient's weight, then the patient should be considered fully dependent and an assistive device should be used. (Waters, T. [2007]. When is it safe to manually lift a patient? *American Journal of Nursing*, 107(8), 40-45.)

A.18

Algorithm 18: Ambulation

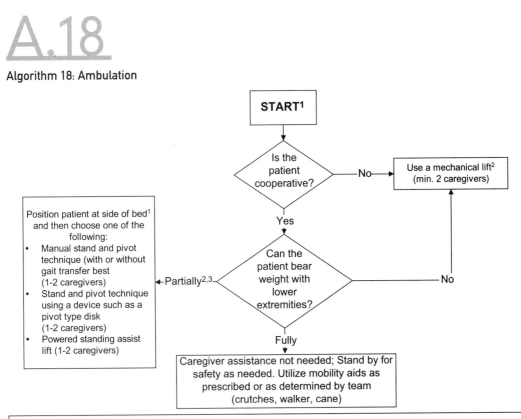

START[1]

Is the patient cooperative? —No→ Use a mechanical lift[2] (min. 2 caregivers)

↓ Yes

Can the patient bear weight with lower extremities? —No→

←Partially[2,3]—

Position patient at side of bed[1] and then choose one of the following:
- Manual stand and pivot technique (with or without gait transfer best (1-2 caregivers)
- Stand and pivot technique using a device such as a pivot type disk (1-2 caregivers)
- Powered standing assist lift (1-2 caregivers)

↓ Fully

Caregiver assistance not needed; Stand by for safety as needed. Utilize mobility aids as prescribed or as determined by team (crutches, walker, cane)

FOOTNOTES:
1. Moving from supine head of bed elevated to setting at edge of bed requires a patient's ability to shift their seated weight in a sitting position:
a. When assistance is not required, this is typically accomplished by unweighting one buttock and moving it toward the edge of the bed; repeating this in alternating fashion, until patient is sitting at the edge of the bed.
b. With an impaired UE or LE:
- if the amount of assistance from caregiver does not exceed 35 lbs., caregiver may provide limb support while patient moves unassisted to side of bed (see a. above)
- if the amount of assistance from caregiver may exceed 35 lbs., then a limb support strap/sling with a mechanical lift will provide limb support while patient moves unassisted to side of bed (see a. above)
c. If patient is unable to accomplish a. and/or b. then utilize one of the following options:
- mechanical lift device with a seated sling to lift patient to side of bed
- friction reducing device to assist staff in pulling patient to side of bed.
d. Friction reducing devices and seated discs may be useful when the amount of caregiver assistance is close to recommended limits, but be aware of skin shearing risks. Shearing is caused when there are two forces moving in opposite directions adjacent to each other (like scissors).
2. Select sling to meet and maintain the patient's pre-op or post-op positioning guideline/precautions for the affected limb/body part(s).
For more information on sling selection, see the "Slings Toolkit" at http://www.visn8.med.va.gov/patientsafetycenter/safePtHandling
3. Patient can bear weight on one leg only (e.g., weight bearing on unaffected limb or limited weight bearing on affected limb).

GENERAL NOTES:
- Need to test the fit of the sling with an immobilized leg.
- Maintain affected extremity immobilization/alignment.
- Use lift device with limb sling if applicable.
- During any patient handling task, if the caregiver is required to lift more than 35 lbs./(16 kg.) of a patient's weight, then the patient should be considered fully dependent and an assistive device should be used. (Waters, T. [2007]. When is it safe to manually lift a patient? *American Journal of Nursing*, 107(8), 40-45.)

Clinical Tool #1: Lifting and Holding Legs or Arms in an Orthopaedic Setting

Introduction

Often when orthopaedic care is being provided, the care giver must lift and/or hold a limb in place while some type of treatment is being provided, such as cast application. It is assumed that you are maintaining a neutral (upright) body posture (not fully flexed); adjust the height of the table. When a caregiver must lift a leg or arm, it is important to make sure that the weight of the limb being lifted does not exceed the strength capability of the caregiver. An ergonomic tool has been developed to assist caregivers in determining whether a specific lift and/or hold of a limb is acceptable and whether some type of lift or hold assist device is needed. For lifts of limbs with casts, an alternate method is presented for assessing whether the lift is acceptable or not as presented in Table #A.1.

This tool shows the calculation of the average weight for an adult patient's leg and arm as a function of whole body mass, ranging from slim to morbidly obese body type. Weights are presented both in pounds (lbs.) and metric (kg.) units. Maximum lift and hold loads were calculated based on 75th percentile shoulder flexion strength and endurance capability for US adult females, where the maximum weight for a one-handed lift is 11.1 lbs. and a two-handed lift, 22.2lbs.

The shaded areas of the table indicate whether it would be acceptable for one caregiver to lift the listed body parts with one or two hands or hold the respective body parts for 1, 2, or 3 minutes with two hands. Respecting these limits will minimize risk of muscle fatigue and the potential for musculoskeletal disorders. If the limb weight exceeds the values listed in the table it is recommended to use assistive technology, such as a ceiling lift or floor based lift with a limb support sling. Orthopaedic caregivers must use clinical judgment to assess the need for additional staff member assistance or assistive devices to lift and/ or hold one of these body parts for a particular period of time.

Note: It is important to remember that the chart shows the acceptable weights for limbs without a cast in place. If the caregiver is lifting a limb with a cast, the additional weight of the cast should be added to the weight of the limb to determine whether the lift is acceptable. An alternate method is provided below for limbs with casts. These are guidelines for the average weight of the leg and arm, and are based upon the patient's weight. The maximum weight for a 1- handed lift is 11.1 lbs. and a 2- handed lift, 22.2 lbs.

Patient weight is divided into weight categories (see Table A.1), ranging from very light to morbidly obese. Normalized weight for each leg and each arm are calculated as a percentage of body weight where each complete arm weighs 5.1% of total body mass and each leg weighs 15.7% of total body mass (Chaffin, Anderson, & Martin, 1999). All weights are presented in both pounds and kilograms, rounded to the nearest whole unit.

To accommodate 75% of the US adult female working population, maximum load for a 1- handed lift is calculated to be 11.1 lbs. (5.0 kg.). This is determined by calculating the strength capabilities for 25th percentile US adult female maximum shoulder flexion movement (the mean equals 40 Newton meters, standard deviation equals 13 Nm) (Chaffin, Anderson, & Martin, 1999) and 75th percentile

Ergonomic Tool: Lifting and Holding Legs or Arms in an Orthopaedic Setting*

Patient Weight lbs. (kg.)	Body Part	Body Part Weight Lbs. (kg.)	Lift 1-hand	Lift 2-hand	Hold 2-hand 1 min.	Hold 2-hand 2 min.	Hold 2-hand 3 min.
<40 lbs. (<18 kg.)	Leg	<6.3 lbs. (3 kg.)					
	Arm	<2.0 lbs. (1 kg.)					
40–90 lbs. (18–41 kg.)	Leg	<14.1 lbs. (6 kg.)					
	Arm	<4.6 lbs. (2 kg.)					
90–140 lbs. (41–64 kg.)	Leg	<22.0 lbs. (10 kg.)					
	Arm	<7.1 lbs. (3 kg.)					
140–190 lbs. (64–86 kg.)	Leg	<29.8 lbs. (14 kg.)					
	Arm	<9.7 lbs. (4 kg.)					
190–240 lbs. (86–109 kg.)	Leg	<37.7 lbs. (17 kg.)					
	Arm	<12.2 lbs. (6 kg.)					
240–290 lbs. (109–132 kg.)	Leg	<45.5 lbs. (21 kg.)					
	Arm	<14.8 lbs. (7 kg.)					
290–340 lbs. (132–155 kg.)	Leg	<53.4 lbs. (24 kg.)					
	Arm	<17.3 lbs. (8 kg.)					
340–390 lbs. (155–177 kg.)	Leg	<61.2 lbs. (28 kg.)					
	Arm	<19.9 lbs. (9 kg.)					
390–440 lbs. (177–200 kg.)	Leg	<69.1 lbs. (31 kg.)					
	Arm	<22.2 lbs. (10 kg.)					
>440 lbs. (>200 kg.)	Leg	>69.1 lbs. (31 kg.)					
	Arm	>22.2 lbs. (10 kg.)					

*No shading: Lift and hold is appropriate but use clinical judgment and do not hold longer than noted: Heavy shading: Do not lift alone: use assistive device or more than 1 caregiver.

US adult female shoulder to grip length (the mean equals 610 mm, the standard deviation equals 30 mm) (Pheasant, 1992). Maximum loads for one person for a 2-handed lift (i.e., 22.2 lbs./10.1 kg.) are calculated as twice that of a 1-handed lift. Muscle strength capabilities diminish as a function of time, therefore, maximum loads for 2-handed holding of body parts are presented for 1, 2, and 3 minute durations. After 1 minute, muscle endurance has decreased by 48%, decreased by 65% after 2 minutes, and, after 3 minutes of continuous holding, strength capability is only 29% of initial lifting strength (Rohmert, 1973, a, b). If the limits in ergonomic Table A.1 are exceeded, additional staff members or assistive limb holders should be used.

References

Chaffin, D. B., Anderson, G.B.J., & Martin, B.J. (1999). *Occupational biomechanics* (3rd ed.). New York, NY: J. Wiley & Sons

Pheasant, S. (1992). *Bodyspace*. Taylor & Francis, Ltd: London.

Rohmert, W. (1973a). Problems of determination of rest allowances. Part 1: Use of modern methods to evaluate stress and strain in static muscular work. *Applied Ergonomics, 4*(2), 91–95.

Rohmert, W. (1973b) Problems of determination of rest allowances. Part 2: Determining rest allowances in different human tasks. *Applied Ergonomics, 4*(3), 158–162.

Waters, T. (2007). When is it safe to manually lift a patient? *American Journal of Nursing, 107*(8), 53–59.

Clinical Tool #2: Alternate Method for Determining Safe Lifting and Holding of Limbs with Casts

A.2 Predicted Weight for Different Types of Casts						
Limb	Limb Weight Factor	1-hand	2-hand	2-hand 1 min.	2-hand 2 min.	2-hand 3 min.
Leg	0.157	11.1 lbs.	22.2 lbs.	11.6 lbs.	7.8 lbs.	6.4 lbs.
Arm	0.051	(5.1 kg.)	(10.2 kg.)	(5.3 kg.)	(3.5 kg.)	(2.9 kg.)

Multiply the patients' weight times the limb factor (0.157 for leg and 0.051 for arm) and add the weight of the cast. Compare the calculated weight to the value in the appropriate task box. If the total limb weight exceeds the weight in the appropriate box, then the caregiver should not manually lift the limb alone but should use an assistive device or more than one caregiver to perform the lift. On the other hand, if the calculated weight is less than the value in the appropriate box, then it is acceptable to manually lift and hold the limb and the caregiver should use clinical judgment and not hold longer than noted.

For example if the patient weighs 200 lbs. and has an arm cast weighing 5 lbs., then the total arm weight would be 200 lbs. × 0.051 + 5 lbs., or 15.2 lbs. In this case, the arm should not be lifted with one hand (i.e., 15.2 lbs. > 11.1 lbs.) but could be lifted with two hands (i.e., 15.2 lbs. < 22.2 lbs.), but not held in that position less than a few seconds (15.2 lbs. > 11.6 lbs.). Similarly, if the patient weighs 75 lbs. and has a 5 lb. leg cast, then the total limb weight would be 75 lbs. × 0.157 + 5 lbs., or 16.8 lbs. In this case, it would not be acceptable to lift the limb with one hand (i.e., 16.8 lbs. > 11.1 lbs.), but it would be acceptable to lift it with two hands (i.e., 16.8 lbs. < 22.1 lbs.), but should not be held more than a few seconds (16.8 lbs. > 11.6 lbs.).

The following Table A.3 provides some predicted weights for a fiberglass cast.

A.3	**Predicted Weights for a Fiberglass Cast**				
Short Arm Cast (adult)	**Long Arm Cast (adult)**	**Short Leg Walking Cast (150 lbs. adult)**	**Long Leg Cast (150 lbs. adult)**	**Infant Body Spica 20–30 lbs.**	**Child Body Spica 3–5-yr-old 30–50 lbs.**
0.5 lbs.	1 lbs.	2 lbs.	3.0 lbs.	2 lbs.	4lbs.
2 rolls 3"	1 roll 2" 3 rolls 3"	4 rolls 4"	3 rolls 3" 3 rolls 4"	2 rolls 2" 3 rolls 3"	5 rolls 3" 5 rolls 4"
+ webril*	+ webril*	+ webril*	+ webril*	+ webril*	+ webril*

*Weight of webril is 0.25 lb. per packet

Notes to Algorithms and Clinical Tools for Safe Patient Handling in an Orthopaedic Setting: Helpful Hints on Slings

Selection of the appropriate sling accessory for movement/lift/transfer, must include the following considerations:

- Decision to transfer patient in sitting vs. supine position – choose correct functionality of the sling
- Select appropriate size
- Maintain alignment of the affected body part(s) according to pre-operative/post-operative guidelines
  - ◆ Consider the patient's body size, shape and features (e.g. very large abdominal girth can limit degree of hip flexion
  - ◆ Features of sling:
    - consider where material covers the patient
    - strap options for seated slings-the length of material for strap supports of the lower extremities can often be modified by selecting differing loop attachment points of the sling onto the hanger bar (e.g. providing more material length will allow lower extremity to be in less flexed position)
    - seated slings back height can vary from supporting whole trunk and head to covering pelvis/waist only. When upper extremities are involved, consider height of the sling – high back slings will wrap around and enclose an upper extremity, while a low back sling will allow upper extremity to be free
- If alignment/positioning guidelines cannot be met with available sling accessory, transfer patient supine with sheet style sling or anti-friction methods, then sit upright.
- The "Patient Care Sling Selection and Usage Toolkit" is available for download at: http://www.visn8.med.va.gov/patientsafetycenter/safePtHandling/toolkitSlings.asp

A.19

Algorithm 19: Lateral Transfer from Stretcher to and from the OR Bed

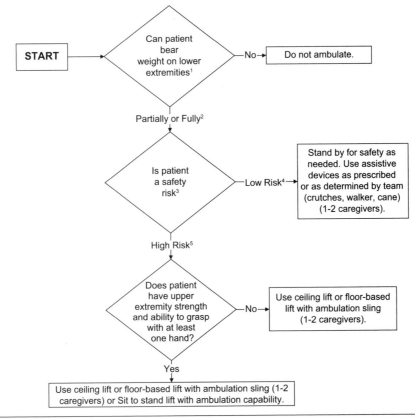

START → Can patient bear weight on lower extremities[1] — No → Do not ambulate.

Partially or Fully[2] ↓

Is patient a safety risk[3] — Low Risk[4] → Stand by for safety as needed. Use assistive devices as prescribed or as determined by team (crutches, walker, cane) (1-2 caregivers).

High Risk[5] ↓

Does patient have upper extremity strength and ability to grasp with at least one hand? — No → Use ceiling lift or floor-based lift with ambulation sling (1-2 caregivers).

Yes ↓

Use ceiling lift or floor-based lift with ambulation sling (1-2 caregivers) or Sit to stand lift with ambulation capability.

FOOTNOTES:
1. Non-weight bearing: Patient is unable to bear weight through both lower extremities or weight bearing through both lower extremities is contraindicated.
2. Partial weight bearing: This will include situations where the patient may be allowed: a) Limited weight bearing on one lower extremity and full weight bearing on the other extremity; b) Partial weight bearing through both lower extremities.
3. Safety risks may include: decreased cognition; decreased ability to cooperate/ combativeness; medical stability.
4. Factors that contribute to low safety risk: a) Lack of combativeness; b) Ability to follow commands; c) Medical stability; d) Experience with the assistive device.
5. Factors that contribute to high safety risk: a) Combativeness; b) Lack of ability to follow commands; c) Medical instability; d) Lack of experience with the assistive device, e) neurological deficits.

GENERAL COMMENTS/DISCUSSION:
- In healthcare, weight bearing is often used to describe the amount of weight bearing that the patient can or has done. In orthopaedics, weight bearing status is prescribed by the physician based on the patient's ability to safely bear weight through the musculoskeletal. Exceeding the prescribed weight bearing status may be detrimental to the patient.
- Patients should be assessed for safety risks as described above. If patients are determined to be at significant risk for falls, then care givers assisting with ambulation are also at risk for assisting patients to prevent fall. In high risk situations precautions should be taken, and devices such as walking slings should be used. At some point in care, the team will need to weigh the risks of falls with the benefits of ambulation and take a "therapeutic" risk in order to functionally advance the patient.
- Need to test the fit of the sling with an immobilized leg. For more informaiton on on sling selection, see the "Slings Toolkit" at http://www.visn8.med.va.gov/safePtHandling
- Maintain affected extremity immobilization/alignment.
- During any patient handling task, if the caregiver is required to lift more than 35 lbs./(16 kg.) of a patient's weight, then the patient should be considered fully dependent and an assistive device should be used. (Waters, T. [2007]. When is it safe to manually lift a patient? *American Journal of Nursing,107* (8), 40-45.)

A.20

Algorithm 20: Positioning and Repositioning the Patient on the OR Bed to and from the Supine Position

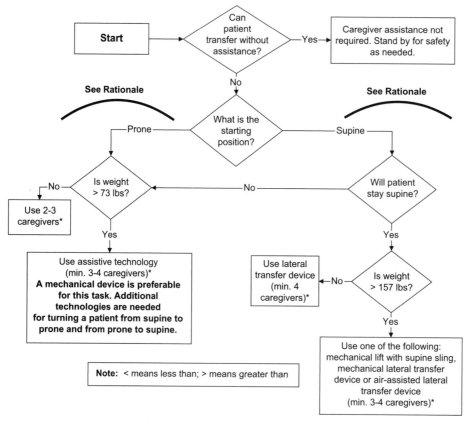

Note: < means less than; > means greater than

- * One of the caregivers may be the anesthesia provider
- The number of personnel to safely transfer the patient should be adequate to maintain the patient's body alignment, support extremities, and maintain patient's airway.
- For lateral transfers it is important to use a lateral transfer device that extends the length of the patient.
- Current technologies for supine to prone include: Jackson Frame, Spine Table, etc.
- Destination surface should be slightly lower for all lateral patient moves.
- A separate algorithm for prone to jackknife is not included as this is assumed to be a function of the table.
- If patient's condition will not tolerate a lateral transfer, consider the use of a mechanical lift with a supine sling.
- During any patient transferring task, if any caregiver is required to lift more than 35 lbs of a patient's weight, assistive devices should be used for the transfer.
- While some facilities may attempt to perform a lateral transfer simultaneously with positioning the patient in a lateral position (ie, side-lying), this is not recommended until new technology is available.
- The assumption is that the patient will leave the operating room in the supine position.

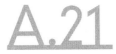

Algorithm 21: Lifting and Holding Legs, Arms, and Heads for Prepping in a Perioperative Setting

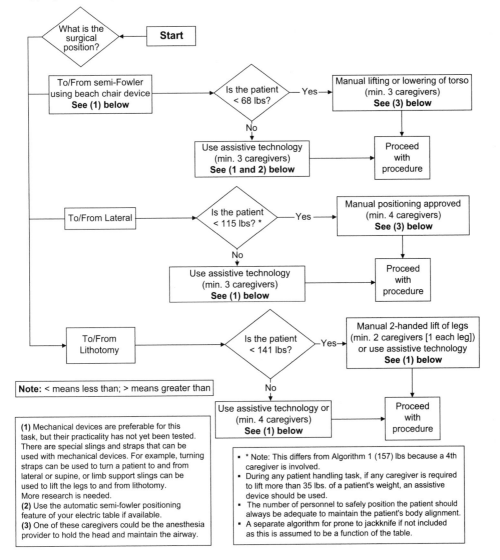

Note: < means less than; > means greater than

(1) Mechanical devices are preferable for this task, but their practicality has not yet been tested. There are special slings and straps that can be used with mechanical devices. For example, turning straps can be used to turn a patient to and from lateral or supine, or limb support slings can be used to lift the legs to and from lithotomy. More research is needed.
(2) Use the automatic semi-fowler positioning feature of your electric table if available.
(3) One of these caregivers could be the anesthesia provider to hold the head and maintain the airway.

- * Note: This differs from Algorithm 1 (157) lbs because a 4th caregiver is involved.
- During any patient handling task, if any caregiver is required to lift more than 35 lbs. of a patient's weight, an assistive device should be used.
- The number of personnel to safely position the patient should always be adequate to maintain the patient's body alignment.
- A separate algorithm for prone to jackknife if not included as this is assumed to be a function of the table.

A.4 Lifting and Holding Legs, Arms, and Heads for Prepping in a Perioperative Setting

Key

No shading	OK to lift and hold: use clinical judgment; do not hold longer than noted
Heavy shading	Do not lift alone: use assistive device or more than one caregiver

(Cells marked ▒ = heavy shading)

Patient Weight lbs (kg)	Body Part	Body Part Weight lbs (kg)	Lift 1-hand	Lift 2-hand	Hold 2-hand ≤1 min	Hold 2-hand ≤2 min	Hold 2-hand ≤3 min
≤120 lbs (≤ 54 kg)	Leg	≤19 lbs (9 kg)	▒			▒	▒
	Arm	≤6 lbs (3 kg)					
	Head	≤10 lbs (5 kg)					▒
120–160 lbs (54–73 kg)	Leg	≤25 lbs (11 kg)	▒		▒	▒	▒
	Arm	≤8 lbs (4 kg)					
	Head	≤13 lbs (6 kg)	▒				
160–200 lbs (73–91 kg)	Leg	≤31 lbs (14 kg)	▒		▒	▒	▒
	Arm	≤10 lbs (5 kg)					
	Head	≤17 lbs (8 kg)	▒				▒
200–240 lbs (91–109 kg)	Leg	≤38 lbs (17 kg)	▒		▒	▒	▒
	Arm	≤12 lbs (6 kg)	▒				
	Head	≤20 lbs (9 kg)	▒			▒	▒
240–280 lbs (109–127 kg)	Leg	≤44 lbs (20 kg)	▒		▒	▒	▒
	Arm	≤14 lbs (6 kg)	▒				▒
	Head	≤24 lbs (11 kg)	▒			▒	▒
280–320 lbs (127–145 kg)	Leg	≤50 lbs (23 kg)	▒	▒	▒	▒	▒
	Arm	≤16 lbs (7 kg)	▒				▒
	Head	≤27 lbs (12 kg)	▒		▒	▒	▒
>360 lbs (>163 kg)	Leg	≥57 lbs (26 kg)	▒	▒	▒	▒	▒
	Arm	≥18 lbs (8 kg)	▒			▒	▒
	Head	≥30 lbs (14 kg)	▒		▒	▒	▒

A.22

Algorithm 22: Prolonged Standing

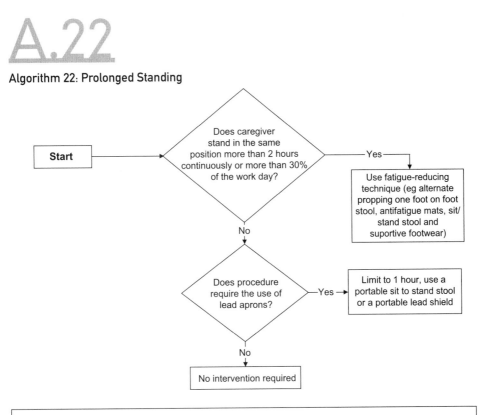

Start

Does caregiver stand in the same position more than 2 hours continuously or more than 30% of the work day?

Yes → Use fatigue-reducing technique (eg alternate propping one foot on foot stool, antifatigue mats, sit/stand stool and suportive footwear)

No

Does procedure require the use of lead aprons?

Yes → Limit to 1 hour, use a portable sit to stand stool or a portable lead shield

No

No intervention required

GENERAL RECOMMENDATIONS

- Caregivers should wear supportive footwear that has the following properties: does not change the shape of the foot; has enough space to move toes; shock-absorbing cushioned insoles; closed toe; height of heel in proportion to the shoe.
- Caregivers may benefit from wearing support stockings/socks.
- Anti-fatigue mats should be on the floors.
- Anti-fatigue mats should be placed on standing stools
- The sit-stand chair should be set to the correct height before setting the sterile field so they will not be changing levels during the procedure.*
- Be aware of infection control issues for non-disposable and anti-fatigue matting.
- The 2-hour limit on prolonged standing incorporates accommodations for pregnancy.
- Scrubbed staff should not work with the neck flexed more than 30 degrees or rotated for more than one minute uninterrupted.
- 2-piece lightweight lead aprons are recommended.
- During the sit-to-stand break, staff should look straight ahead for a short while.

---

* "AORN Recommended practices for maintaining a sterile field," in *Standards, Recommended Practices, and Guidelines* (Denver: AORN, Inc, 2006) 621-628.

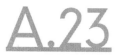

Algorithm 23: Retraction

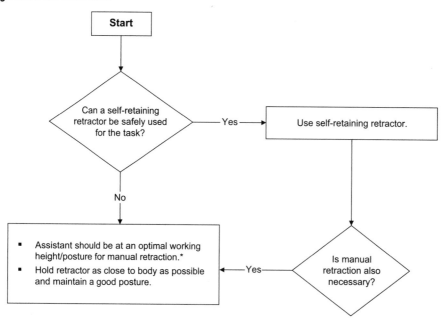

---

* Optimal working height is defined as area between the chest and the waist height to operative field. Optimal posture is defined as perpendicular/straight-on to the operative field; asymmetrical posture may be acceptable depending on load and duration; torso twisting should be avoided at all times.

- Arm rests should be used as possible, and be large enough to allow repositioning of the arms.
- Under optimal working height and posture, an assistive device should be used to lift or hold more than 35 lbs.
- Further research is needed to determine time limits for exposure. This is a high risk task, therefore, team members should take rest breaks or reposition when possible.
- Avoid using the hands as an approach to retraction, it is very high risk for musculoskeletal or sharps injuries.

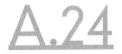

Algorithm 24: Lifting and Carrying Supplies and Equipment

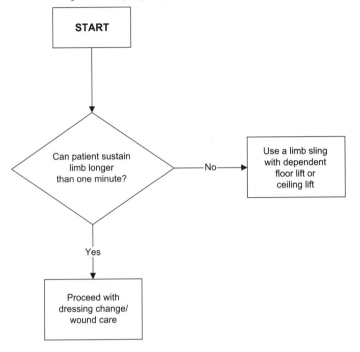

GENERAL NOTES:

- For any patient who has, or is at risk for a pressure ulcer, care should be taken to avoid shearing force (such as using a friction reducing device for repositioning in bed).
- The height of the bed should be appropriate for staff safety (at elbow height).
- During any patient handling task, if the caregiver is required to lift more than 35 lbs./16 kg. of a patient's weight, then the patient should be considered fully dependent and an assistive device should be used. (Waters, T. [2007]. When is it safe to manually lift a patient? *American Journal of Nursing, 107*(8), 40-45.)

A.5 Ergonomic Risks: Lifting

Lifting Task	Lifting Index	Level of Risk
3000 ml irrigation fluid	<0.2	
Sand bags	0.3	
Linen bags	0.4	
Lead aprons	0.4	
Custom sterile packs (e.g., heart or spine)	0.5	
Garbage bags (full)	0.7	
Positioning devices off shelf or rack (e.g., stirrups)	0.7	
Positioning devices off shelf or rack (e.g., gel pads)	0.9	
Hand table (49" X 28")—largest hand table—used infrequently	1.2	(light shading)
Fluoroscopy Board (49" X 21")	1.2	(light shading)
Stirrups (2—one in each hand)	1.4	(light shading)
Wilson frame	1.4	(light shading)
Irrigation containers for lithotripsy (12,000 ml)	1.5	(light shading)
Instrument pans	2.0	(heavy shading)

Key

No shading	Minimal risk—Safe to lift
Light shading	Potential risk—Use assistive technology, as available
Heavy shading	Considerable risk—One person should not perform alone or weight should be reduced

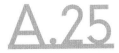

Algorithm 25: Pushing, Pulling and Moving Equipment on Wheels

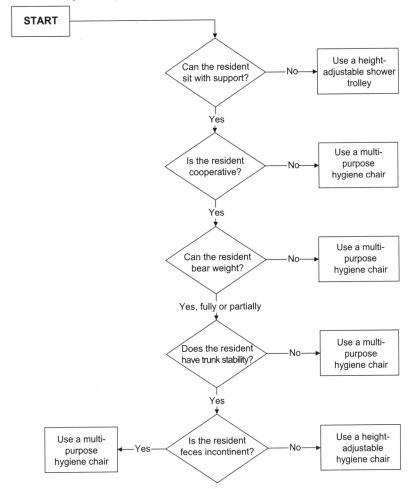

GENERAL NOTES:
- For any patient who has, or is at risk for a pressure ulcer, care should be taken to avoid shearing force (such as using a friction reducing device for repositioning in bed).
- The height of the bed should be appropriate for staff safety (at elbow height).
- During any patient handling task, if the caregiver is required to lift more than 35 lbs./16 kg. of a patient's weight, then the patient should be considered fully dependent and an assistive device should be used. (Waters, T. [2007]. When is it safe to manually lift a patient? *American Journal of Nursing, 107* (8), 40-45.)

A.6 Ergonomic Risks: Movement of OR Equipment

OR Equipment	Pushing Force lbF (kgF)		Max Push Distance ft/s (m)		Ergonomic Recommendation
Electrosurgery unit	8.4 lbF	(3.8 kgF)	>200 ft	(60 m)	Task is acceptable for 1 caregiver
Ultrasound	12.4 lbF	(5.6 kgF)	>200 ft	(60 m)	
X ray equipment portable	12.9 lbF	(5.9 kgF)	>200 ft	(60 m)	
Video towers	14.1 lbF	(6.4 kgF)	>200 ft	(60 m)	
Linen cart	16.3 lbF	(7.4 kgF)	>200 ft	(60 m)	
X ray equip—C-arm	19.6 lbF	(8.9 kgF)	>200 ft	(60 m)	
Case carts—empty	24.2 lbF	(11.0 kgF)	>200 ft	(60 m)	
OR stretcher unoccupied	25.1 lbF	(11.4 kgF)	>200 ft	(60 m)	
Case carts—full	26.6 lbF	(12.1 kgF)	>200 ft	(60 m)	
Microscopes	27.5 lbF	(12.5 kgF)	>200 ft	(60 m)	
Hospital bed—unoccupied	29.8 lbF	(13.5 kgF)	>200 ft	(60 m)	
Specialty equip carts	39.3 lbF	(17.9 kgF)	>200 ft	(60 m)	
OR stretcher—occupied 300 lbs	43.8 lbF	(19.9 kgF)	>200 ft	(60 m)	
Bed—occupied 300 lbs	50.0 lbF	(22.7 kgF)	<200 ft	(30 m)	Min 2 caregivers required
Specialty OR beds unoccupied	69.7 lbF	(31.7 kgF)	<100 ft	(30 m)	
OR bed unoccupied	61.3 lbF	(27.9 kgF)	<25 ft	(7.5 m)	Recommend powered transport device
OR bed occupied 300 lbs	112.4 lbF	(51.1 kgF)	<25 ft	(7.5 m)	
Specialty OR beds—occupied 300 lbs	124.2 lbF	(56.5 kgF)	<25 ft	(7.5 m)	

Key

No shading	Minimal risk—Task is acceptable for 1 caregiver
Light shading	Moderate risk—Minimum of 2 caregivers or powered device recommended
Heavy shading	Considerable risk—Recommend powered transport device

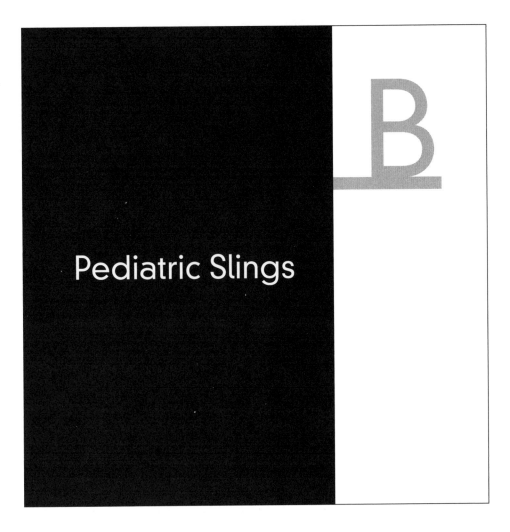

Pediatric Slings

Guldmann Slings

		Kids 4–6	Kids 6–10	Kids 10–14
↕	Height* (inches)	18 1/8 – 23 5/8	21 5/8 – 30 3/8	26 6/8 – 31 4/8
↔	Width* (inches)	9 7/8 – 11 6/8	11 – 13 6/8	13 – 15

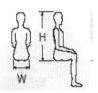

* Choose sling size primarily based on width measurements vs. height measurements.
Width should be measured between the widest points across the hips/buttocks (vs. using the hip bones/ASIS).

Guldmann Slings *(Continued)*

	XS	S	M	L	XL	XXL	XXXL
Height* (inches)	29 4/8 – 32 2/8	31 4/8 – 34 2/8	33 4/8 – 36 2/8	35 3/8 – 38 2/8	37 3/8 – 40 1/8	37 3/8 – 40 1/8	37 3/8 – 40 1/8
Width* (inches)	13 – 14 5/8	14 1/8 – 15 6/8	15 3/8 – 16 7/8	16 4/8 – 17 6/8	17 6/8 – 19 2/8	17 7/8 – 20 4/8	21 2/8 – 22 7/8

*Choose sling size primarily based on width measurements vs. height measurements.
Width should be measured between the widest points across the hips/buttocks (vs. using the hip bones/ASIS).

Max lifting capacity for all Guldmann ABC slings: 250 kg		Size									
		Kids 4–6	Kids 6–10	Kids 10–14	XS	S	M	L	XL	XXL	XXXL
ACTIVE											
Micro plus	polyester	281001	281011	281021							
Micro plus	polyester				281531	281541	281551	281561	281571	281581	
Trainer	polyester	283001	283011	283021	283031	283041	283051	283061	283071	283081	
BASIC											
Basic	polyester	270001	270011	270021	270031	270041	270051	270061	270071	270081	
Basic	net	270102	270112	270122	270132	270142	270152	270162	270172	270182	
Basic Low	polyester				271031	271041	271051	271061	271071	271081	
Basic Low	net				271132	271142	271152	271162	271172	271182	
Basic High	polyester	272001	272011	272021	272031	272041	272051	272061	272071	272081	
Basic High*	polyester										273031
Basic High	net	272102	272112	272122	272132	272142	272152	272162	272172	272182	
CUSTOM											
Amputee	polyester					290041	290051	290061			
Sit-On**	net						291052		291082		
Sit-On**	net						292052		292082		

* Basic High XXL lift up to 1,000 lbs.
** Sit-On slings are available in two all –size models: Standard and Wide

For reference: http://www.guldmann.com

Arjo/Huntleigh Pediatric Slings

	Size	Color	Weight Range
Pediatrics	XXS	Teal	0–25 kg (0–55 lbs)
	XS	Brown	25–35 kg (55–77 lbs)
Adults	S	Red	35–60 kg (77–132 lbs)
	M	Yellow	55–75 kg (121–165 lbs)
	L	Green	70–120 kg (154–264 lbs)
	LL	Purple	100–160 kg (220–350 lbs)
	XL	Blue	140–200 kg (308–440 lbs)
	XXL	Terracotta	200–228 kg (440–500 lbs)
Bariatric	Bariatric M	Yellow/Dark Gray	160–210 kg (350–450 lbs)
	Bariatric L	Green/Dark Gray	210–250 kg (450–555 lbs)
	Bariatric XL	Blue/Dark Gray	230–340 kg (500–750 lbs)
	Bariatric XXL	Terracotta/Dark Gray	318–455 kg (700–1000 lbs)

	Size	Length from Tailbone to Upper Point of Head
Pediatrics	XXS	43–52 cm
	XS	52–61 cm
	S	61–73 cm
	M	73–85 cm
	L	85–95 cm
	LL	95–100 cm
	XL	100–105 cm
	XXL	105–115 cm

For reference: http://www.arjohuntleigh.com

Liko Pediatric Slings

Teddy Slings for Playful Lifting

Children are not miniature adults. Lifting children requires extra care and specially adapted accessories. Over the years, Liko has developed a full range of specially adapted accessories for lifting children. Now, Liko has added an important feature—children's slings with a teddy bear motif.

The new Teddy Slings, in a soft warp-knitted polyester with a teddy bear pattern, have become a great success. Teddy slings are available in 10 functional models for varying needs and lifting situations. They are complemented by Liko's other children's slings in different net fabrics for sitting shell and shower/bath situations.

In addition to the world's most complete range of slings, Liko now has the most play-friendly slings for playful children.

Teddy Pants

Application area: Lift pants in Teddy fabric make gait training not only safe, but fun. Kids love to hop around in Teddy Pants.

Design features: Padded with synthetic sheepskin around the stomach and crotch. Padding bases are available as an accessory (Part No. 3666021).

Sizes: Mod. 92, XS (Part No. 3592823).

Teddy Vest

Application area: The Teddy Vest adapts to the child's physique, lifting around the upper body just enough to allow the child to stand and support his/her weight, according to his/her capability.

Design features: Teddy Vests are available in two models: Mod. 60 and 64. Mod. 64 is equipped with safety clasps for variable width adjustment. Leg Harness (Part No. 3666004) available as an accessory.

Sizes: Mod. 60, XS (Part No. 3560813); Mod. 60, XXS (Part No. 3560812); Mod. 64, XS (Part NO. 3564813)

Teddy Sling Highback

Application area: Teddy Sling Highback allows a comfortable reclined sitting posture with support for the head. Can be used for all lifting to and from horizontal or seated positions. Perfect for lifting to and from the floor. Children with spasticity problems usually sit quite well in Mod. 26. This model is available in other fabrics and versions.

Design features: Reinforced back, head and leg supports. Belt with safety clasps.

Sizes: Mod. 26, Small (Part No. 3526814); Mod. 26, XS (Part No. 3526813)

Silhouette Sling

Application area: We developed the Silhouette Sling especially for children who sit in molded seats and therefore require a sling that can be left in the chair after the transfer. The child's arms can be held either inside or outside the sling.

Design features: Sewn in a thin, pliable polyester net fabric that allows water to pass through.

Sizes: Mod. 22, Small (Part No. 3522604); Mod. 22, XS, (Part No. 3522603)

Teddy Sling Low

Application area: Teddy Sling Low is ideal for lifting to and from sitting/ semi-sitting positions or floor, if the child requires no extra support for the head. This model is available in other fabrics and versions.

Design features: Reinforcement in back and leg supports. Belt with safety clasps.

Sizes: Mod. 10, Small (Part No. 3510864)

Teddy HygieneVest

Application area: Teddy HygieneVest is designed for lifting to and from the toilet, but is ideal for many other lifting situations where you want to achieve an upright and stable sitting posture. This vest lifts around the upper body, which inhibits the tendency to slouch. Children with spasticity problems usually sit quite well in Mod. 55.

Design features: Reinforced leg supports. Model 55 has head support.

Sizes: Mod. 50, XS (Part No. 3550813); Mod. 50, XXS (Part No. 3550812); Mod. 55, XS (Part No. 35558123); Mod. 55, XXS (Part No. 3555812)

Teddy Hygiene Sling

Application area: Teddy Hygiene Sling is designed for lifting to and from the toilet, but is ideal for many other lifting situations.

Design features: Soft padding under the arms and reinforced leg supports. Mo. 41 is equipped with a belt, and Mod. 46 has a Security Belt for added safety, as well as extra back support for optimal comfort.

Sizes: Mod. 41, XS (Part No. 3541813); Mod. 46, XS (Part No. 3546813)

Teddy Vest for Standing Shell

Application area: We have designed the Vest for Standing Shell for the often-difficult lifting situation where a child in a standing shell has to be raised from the floor to a standing position. The lift takes all the weight and the child is lifted safely and comfortably with support for the entire body and head.

Design features: Head support and padded Leg Harness included.

Sizes: Mod. 67, Small (Part No. 3567814); Mod. 67, XS (Part NO. 3567813)

For reference: http://www.liko.com/na

Glossary

Term	Definition
Algorithm	A step-by-step decision map for solving a problem in a finite number of steps. Algorithms that have been developed for safe patient handling progress though a series of decision boxes to determine which technology and how many caregivers are needed to perform the task safely. Algorithms are to be used as a guide and should not replace good clinical judgment. Algorithms offer an advantage of reducing unnecessary variations in practice likely to affect patient and caregiver outcomes. See Appendix A.
Ambulation	Functional capacity to walk from place to place or move about. Ambulation can be independent or partially assisted, with or without the use of assistive devices such as canes, crutches, walkers, wheelchairs, scooters, orthotics, or prosthetics. Ambulation is considered to be a risky task for the patient and the caregiver if the patient is assessed to be at high risk for falls.
Awkward Posture	Awkward positioning of the caregiver's body while performing patient-handling tasks that may increase risk for injury. It is generally considered that the more a joint deviates from the neutral (natural) position, the greater the risk of injury. The longer the duration of the awkward posture, the higher the risk. Examples of awkward postures include excessive reaching in front or behind, excessive reaching high or low, and bending/ twisting.
Back Injury Resource Nurse (BIRNS)	See Unit-Based Peer Safety Leaders
Bariatrics	The science of providing health care to patients who fall into one of these categories: ■ Overweight by greater than 100 lbs ■ Body Mass Index (BMI) greater than 40 ■ Total weight exceeds 300 lbs
Barrier Free	Structural design of the built environment to provide full access to persons with disabilities.
Body Jacket	An apparatus used for alignment of the trunk of the body. Used for patients with spinal cord injuries and spinal cord dysfunction. Caring for a patient in a full-body jacket presents patient-handling and patient-safety challenges.

Body Mass Index (BMI)	The BMI can be calculated by dividing the patient's weight (in kg) by the patient's height squared (m^2).
Body Mechanics	A system for positioning the caregiver's body during patient handling and movement for optimal mechanical advantage. Good body mechanics was once thought to protect caregivers from musculoskeletal risk, but now evidence supports that body mechanics alone cannot protect a caregiver from a musculoskeletal injury.
Boom	The boom connects the mast of the hoist with the spreader/attachment bar. Generally a longer boom is useful for taller/larger patients as it provides more leg room and reduces the potential for the patient's legs knocking against the mast. A peaked boom will bring the patient closer to the mast as the boom rises, and so care must be taken that the patient's knees do not knock against the mast.
Bowel Program	A plan to set up and institute a daily bowel-evacuation routine for persons with neurogenic bowel. A bowel program includes diet, fluid intake monitoring, chemical and mechanical stimulation of the bowel to establish a routine and to reduce unplanned bowel evacuations.
Care Plan	A patient plan of action that takes into consideration patient assessment. For safe patient handling, the care plan includes type of task to be completed, type of equipment or assistive devices needed, and number of caregivers needed to complete the task safely. See Appendix A.
Caregiver	Patient care providers of any discipline and varying educational levels who provide direct patient care, including patient-handling tasks. Caregivers may work in acute care, long-term care, or outpatient or home-based settings. In acute care, caregivers can work in traditional patient care units/wards or perform caregiving responsibilities in radiology, diagnostic labs, morgues, dental, or other settings where patient transfers and/or patient-handling tasks are needed.
Caregiver Risk	Work-related hazards that contribute to musculoskeletal injury or disorders in persons who provide direct patient care.
Ceiling-Mounted Patient Lift	A ceiling lift is a motor that rides on a system of rails permanently affixed to the ceiling or on a mobile gantry with a strap and connection device to apply a sling that can assist in transferring, repositioning, or moving a patient anywhere the rails will allow. Many types of slings are available for performing caregiving tasks.

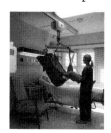 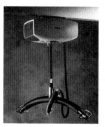 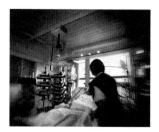

Chairing	Some beds have the capability to position into a "chair position," also known as the cardiac chair position. This bed feature assists the patient to sit upright; the foot of the bed drops down to assist the legs to bend at the knees as in a chair seated position. When the patient requires the health benefits of a seated position, this feature can be used, thus eliminating the need to perform a high-risk patient-transfer task. This bed feature is particularly useful when the patient's tolerance for sitting is limited (e.g., 10–15 minutes) due to pain, fatigue, illness, or disability.
Chassis	The majority of lifts have a U-shaped framework. The chassis height determines if the hoist can go under items of furniture (e.g., bed, chair). Adjustment of the chassis (width between lift legs) may be required to allow the lift to be positioned nearer items of furniture (chairs, beds, etc.) or the patient (e.g., if patient on the floor). The longer the chassis, the more space is required to manoeuvre and position the lift.
Chemical Stimulation	Use of laxatives or enemas to remove stool from the bowel. See also Bowel Program or Neurogenic Bowel.
Cognition	The mental process of knowing, including aspects such as awareness, perception, reasoning, and judgment. Cognition is included as one element of patient-assessment criteria to determine the level of assistance a patient will be able to provide in performing patient-handling tasks.
Compression Stocking Applicator	Device used to don or doff anti-embolism stockings, with less risk to the caregiver.
Compression Stockings	Anti-embolism stockings used for the prevention of deep vein thrombosis (DVT) or for the management of long-term venous insufficiency. Unfortunately, the application or removal of correctly sized stockings is considered a high-risk task because of the high force needed for gripping and the excessive weight lifted and held in awkward positions when applying or removing the stocking.
Cooperation	The level of supportive assistance by a patient in working with a caregiver to complete patient-handling tasks; the level of cooperation can vary over the course of a day and is affected by fatigue, pain, cognition, personality, medications, sleep deprivation, and other factors.
Culture of Safety	Describes the collective attitude of employees taking shared responsibility for safety in a work environment and by doing so, providing a safe environment of care for themselves as well as patients.
Digital Stimulation	A technique that involves insertion of a gloved finger into the rectum to stimulate bowel evacuation in a person with a neurogenic bowel. See also Bowel Program or Neurogenic Bowel.
Electric Profiling Beds	Beds with special features built in to facilitate powered adjustments to patient positioning.
Ergo Coaches	See Unit-Based Peer Safety Leaders.
Ergo Rangers	See Unit-Based Peer Safety Leaders.

Ergonomics	The scientific study of the relation between people and their occupation, equipment, and environment. In simple terms, ergonomics is designing a work environment for human use.
Expanded Capacity (EC)	Equipment designed for bariatric patients are said to have expanded capacity (EC). The exact weight capacity of each type and brand of equipment varies.
Fall-Prevention Program	A plan to reduce the number and severity of patient falls by addressing modifiable risk factors unique to that patient.
Fall Risk	Criteria developed to evaluate and assess a patient's likelihood of a fall. There are several valid and reliable tools to screen for falls and assess for fall risk. Patients deemed to be at high risk for falls increase the caregiver's risk for musculoskeletal injury when engaged in ambulation or transfer tasks.
Floor-Based Patient Lift	These powered, portable lifts need to be transported to the patient room and promote safe patient transfers. Caregivers can also raise a person who has fallen to the floor without needing to sit the patient up first. Some lifts are offered with dual controls, which means the caregiver can choose the most convenient solution for each task by using the handset or the mast control panel. Some offer an adjustable chassis operated from the handset allowing access for patient transfers involving large chairs, wheelchairs, or toilets. Some also have a scale option, with can allow the caregiver to quickly weigh the patient during a transfer. Each manufacturer provides patient slings specific to its lifts. This type of equipment is particularly suited for use in unpredicted situations where a ceiling lift system is not available, e.g., a patient falls in a hallway where ceiling rails are not accessible.

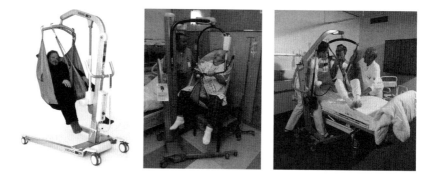

Force	Strength or energy exerted or needed to perform a task.
Friction-Reducing Device (FRD)	A friction-reducing device is a piece of material with a special coating that gives it a very slippery surface. Using these pieces of material (which can be as small as a chair seat or as large as a bed sheet), a caregiver can easily insert a sling behind and under a dependent patient, or slide one on top of the other to easily move a patient horizontally (such as from a bed to a stretcher). These come in many configurations, and some are available with a self-locking material that will keep the patient from sliding down once he or she has been positioned.

Functional Ability	Pertaining to the movement and actions of a part; pertaining to the function of a part, organ, or prosthesis, and whether or not the patient is able to perform the function; function includes physical, cognitive, and emotional capabilities.
Gait	The manner or style of walking.
Height-Adjustable Hygiene Chair	Commode/shower chair that is powered to allow the caregiver to raise the patient to a comfortable height while performing hygiene tasks, such as bathing, dressing, undressing, and changing incontinence pads.
Height-Adjustable Working Stool	A sitting device that can be lowered or made higher to position the caregiver at the optimum height for the task being performed, e.g., feeding a patient.
High Risk Patient-Handling Task	A patient-care activity that has been demonstrated to cause musculoskeletal injuries in caregivers. Tasks are deemed high risk based on a combination of the frequency, duration, and strenuousness of the task.
Hygiene Care	Tasks that can be included in the cleanliness routines (i.e., dressing, undressing, changing incontinence pads, washing certain body parts, full-body showering, hair washing, foot care, and toileting). Patients may be independent in these tasks, may need partial assistance, or may need full assistance from the caregiver.
Incontinence Pad	A flat cloth or disposable material placed under a patient who is unable to control excretory functions.
Infection Control	Preventing or decreasing the invasion and multiplication of microorganisms in body tissues, especially those causing cellular injury due to competitive metabolism, toxins, intracellular replication, or antigen-antibody response; preventing infectious disease.
Kilogram (kg)	The base unit of mass in the International System of Units, equal to 1000 g (2.2 lbs).
Lateral Patient Transfer	Movement of a supine patient from one surface to another, e.g., bed to stretcher, bed to prone cart, or bed to bath trolley.
Lift/Hoist	A lift is a device that can be used to assist the transfer of a patient from one surface to another or to reposition a patient. Lifts are generally operated electrically. There are a variety of designs including portable, mobile, ceiling-mounted, and gantry systems. The most common type of mobile lift features a chassis, mast, boom and spreader bar to which the sling attaches. Lifts must only be used in accordance with manufacturers' instructions, compatible slings, and after patient assessment.
Manual Patient Handling	Lifting, transferring, repositioning, and moving patients using a caregiver's body strength without the use of lifting equipment/aids to reduce forces on the caregiver's musculoskeletal structure. Manual patient handling is performed at high risk to the patient and the caregiver.
Mast	The lift mast is an upright column that connects the chassis with the boom. The height of the mast contributes to the lifting height of the lift. The steering handle of a mobile lift is also attached to the mast.

Minimal-Lift Policy	One evidence-based program element of a comprehensive approach to preventing musculoskeletal injuries in caregivers. The intent of the policy is to establish the minimum standards for safe patient handling by providing written guidelines that can be used by health care administrators, supervisors, and front-line employees to allocate resources and understand and apply the elements of a safe patient-handling program. The basic premise is that manual handling of patients should be avoided wherever possible. (Also referred to as "zero-lift," "no-lift", "no-manual-lift," or "safe-lifting policy.")
Mobility	The functional ability to move readily from place to place, with or without the use of mobility-related assistive devices.
Mobility-Related Assistive Devices	Devices used to facilitate patient functional capabilities to ambulate. Mobility-related assistive devices include, but are not limited to, canes, crutches, walkers, wheelchairs, scooters, orthotics, or prosthetics.
Multipurpose Hygiene Chair	A height adjustable chair that facilitates patient comfort as well as ergonomic patient access when completing tasks such as bathing, toileting or dressing.
Musculoskeletal Disorders (MSDs)	Injuries and disorders of the muscles, nerves, tendons, ligaments, joints, cartilage, and spinal disc; examples include carpal tunnel syndrome, rotator cuff tendonitis, and epicondylitis.
Neurogenic Bowel	The loss of normal bowel function caused by damage to part of the nervous system.
NIOSH (National Institute for Occupational Safety and Health)	In the United States, the research institution that provides scientific data upon which the Occupational Safety and Health Administration (OSHA) makes recommendations for workplace safety.
No-Lift Policy	See Minimal-Lift Policy
No-Manual-Lift Policy	See Minimal-Lift Policy
Occupational Illness	Any abnormal condition or disorder, other than one resulting from an occupational injury, caused by exposure to factors associated with employment. It includes acute and chronic illnesses or diseases that may be caused by inhalation, absorption, ingestion, or direct contact. The broad categories of occupational illnesses are skin diseases and disorders, dust diseases of the lungs, respiratory condition due to toxic agents, poisoning (systemic effects of toxic materials), disorders due to physical agents other than toxic materials, and disorders from repeated trauma.
Occupational Injuries	Any injury such as a cut, fracture, sprain, amputation, etc., which results from a work-related event or from a single, instantaneous exposure in the work environment.

Occupational Safety and Health Administration (OSHA)	In the United States, the mission of the federal government's Occupational Safety and Health Administration (OSHA) is to save lives, prevent injuries, and protect the health of America's workers. Private employers and some state employees are covered by the Occupational Safety and Health Act of 1970.
Pannus	The abdominal mass or skin mass on the bariatric patient. Often caregivers must lift this mass in order to access the perineum or abdominal area for tasks such as hygiene care, skin and wound assessment, or catheter insertion. Skin in this area is often in poor condition and can easily tear. The underside of the pannus may also have excoriation, sores, fungal infections, or inflammation. The skin and body can be in a congested state, causing fluid retention, swelling in tissues, and leakage of fluid through the skin.
Patient Assessment Criteria for Safe Patient Handling	A tool to assist health care workers in considering critical patient characteristics that affect decisions for selecting the safest equipment and techniques for patient-handling and movement tasks. Criteria include the ability of the patient to bear weight; upper-extremity strength of the patient; ability of the patient to cooperate and follow instructions; patient height and weight; special circumstances likely to affect transfer or repositioning; conditions, such as abdominal wounds, contractures, or presence of tubes; specific physician orders or physical therapy recommendations that relate to transferring or repositioning patients. See Appendix A.
Patient-Care Sling	A fabric device that is used with mechanical lifting equipment to temporarily lift or suspend a patient or body part to perform a patient-handling task. A disposable or patient-specific sling is used for one patient only. Slings are designed for ambulation, limb support, or to suspend the patient in a standing, supine, or seated position. See also Appendix B.
Patient-Handling Equipment	Technology solutions for performing high-risk patient-handling tasks. Categories of patient-handling equipment include, but are not limited to, ceiling-mounted patient lifts, floor-based patient lifts, sit-to-stand lifts, lateral-transfer aids, patient-transport devices, and repositioning devices.
Postmortem Care	Care provided to a patient immediately after death, maintaining patient dignity and proper patient body alignment, with minimal occurrence of skin damage or discoloration. Rigor mortis, the stiffening of the deceased muscles, will begin to occur within 2 to 4 hours after death, which may cause difficulty in positioning the body.
Powered Positioning	Allows the caregiver to change a patient's posture using the assistance of the patient-lift system. This technology is available for both floor-based and ceiling-mounted patient lifts.
Prone	Body position characterized by lying on the abdomen and having the face downward.

Repetitive-Motion Injuries	Damage to tendons, nerves, and other soft tissues that is caused by the repeated performance of a limited number of physical movements and is characterized by numbness, pain, and muscle weakness.
Repositioning	Adjusting patient's position in a bed or chair to prevent pressure ulcers and promote comfort.
Risk Factor	Aspect of the work environment that causes or aggravates a work-related musculoskeletal disorder. Risk factors can be environmental (e.g., cramped work spaces), organizational (e.g., policies or staffing levels), personal (e.g., impairments), or task related (e.g., repetitive motion, pushing/pulling).
Safe Patient-Handling Policy	See Minimal-Lift Policy
Safe Patient-Handling Program	An evidence-based approach to reducing risk to caregivers. Includes the following key elements: hazard assessment in the workplace, use of lifting equipment and devices, patient assessment, planning care using algorithms for safe patient handling, unit-based peer safety leaders, and after-action reviews or safety huddles.
Seated Slings	Devices that enable caregivers to transfer and lift patients in a sitting position, reposition patients in a chair, or bathe them, among other uses.
Shearing Force	Strength or energy exerted to cut through an object. Certain patient-handling tasks put patients at risk of skin shearing from this force, for example, when sliding patients from one surface to another or when removing a sling.
Sit-to-Stand Lift	This is a battery-powered patient lift that allows a patient with some upper-body strength but weak lower extremities to be lifted from the seated to standing position for transfer to and from bed, chair, commode, or toilet. The patient places his or her feet on a platform, and a sling is placed around the back and under the underarms. This sling is attached to the lift, and the patient, holding a bar with both hands, if lifted up by the sling.

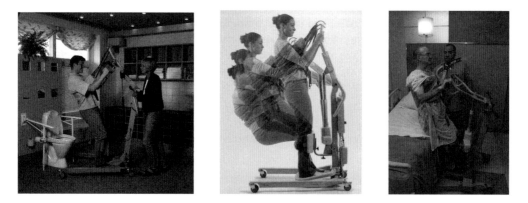

Spinal Loading	The pressure exerted on the spine when performing a patient-handling task. Can refer to compression (downward) or lateral (side or shearing) force on spine.
Spreader Bar/ Attachment Bar	The patient's sling attaches to the lift spreader/attachment bar. Some lifts have interchangeable spreader bars depending upon the type of lift being undertaken (e.g., supine or sitting patient). The design of the spreader bar determines the compatibility of the sling with which it can be used. Most spreader bars can be rotated through 360°; some also feature a tilting design (manual or powered) that aids patient positioning during the transfer.
Stand-Assist Aid	A device that enables patient to transfer from sitting position to standing position.
Static Load	Awkward positioning of the caregiver's body while performing patient-handling tasks that require the caregiver to remain in one place over time. The longer the duration of the static posture, the higher the risk. An example of static load is prolonged standing in one position during a procedure.
Supine	Body position characterized by lying on the back and having the face upward.
Technique	A maneuver, method, or procedure used in safe patient handling.
Torque	A force that produces or tends to produce rotation or torsion; also, a measure of the effectiveness of such a force that consists of the product of the force and the perpendicular distance from the line of action of the force to the axis of rotation; a turning or twisting force. Can produce MSD in caregivers.
Total Hip Replacement Precautions	Safety measures used post-hip replacement surgery, which requires the patient maintain hip abduction, avoid internal rotation, and avoid hip flexion greater than 90 degrees.
Transfer Board	A transfer board is a piece of wood or heavy plastic with high capacity. It is used as a bridge between a chair or commode and bed to allow the patient to slide from one surface to the other without having to stand.
Unit-Based Peer Safety Leaders	Designated direct caregivers responsible for supporting co-workers in providing safe patient care and safe working environments. Their primary role is to coach co-workers in safe patient handling, conduct unit-based hazard assessments, and conduct annual competency evaluations of peers in use of patient-handling equipment. Also known as Back Injury Resource Nurses (BIRNs), Ergo Rangers, or Ergo Coaches.
Unweighting	Removing the heaviness of the body or body part. For example, shifting the caregiver's weight from one foot to another.
U.S. Bureau of Labor Statistics (BLS)	United States governmental agency providing safety and health statistics concerning occupational injuries and illnesses. Widely used as benchmarks by industry, although it uses statistical techniques to extrapolate rates for all employers from a small sample.

U.S. Depart-ment of Labor	United States governmental agency charged with issues relating to workplace safety and health, pensions and benefit plans, employment, and other issues related to the U.S. workplace.
Vertical Transfer	Movement of a patient in a seated position from one surface to another, e.g., bed to wheelchair, bed to chair, chair to toilet, wheelchair to bed-side chair, or car to wheelchair.
Veterans Health Admin-istration (VHA)	Provides a broad spectrum of medical, surgical, and rehabilitative care to veterans in the United States.
Weight Capacity	The maximum number of pounds that can be lifted safely manually, or the manufacturer's documented lifting limits for a specific equip-ment or device. Equipment designed for bariatric patients is said to have "expanded capacity" (EC). The exact weight capacity of each type and brand of equipment varies. See also Expanded Capacity.
Workload	The amount of work assigned to or expected from a worker in a specified time period.
Work-Related Musculoskel-etal Disorders (WRMSD, WMSD)	See Musculoskeletal Disorders (MSDs)
Zero-Lift Policy	See Minimal-Lift Policy

Index

W

V

X